Ethics in Hospice Care: Challenges to Hospice Values in a Changing Health Care Environment

Ethics in Hospice Care: Challenges to Hospice Values in a Changing Health Care Environment

Bruce Jennings, MA
Editor

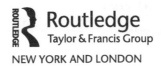

Routledge
Taylor & Francis Group

NEW YORK AND LONDON

First published in 1997 by
The Haworth Press, Inc., 10 Alice Street, Binghamton, NY 13904-1580 USA

Published 2016 by Routledge
711 Third Avenue, New York, NY 10017
2 Park Square, Milton Park, Abingdon, Oxfordshire OX14 4RN

First issued in paperback 2016

Routledge is an imprint of the Taylor and Francis Group, an informa business

Ethics in Hospice Care: Challenges to Hospice Values in a Changing Health Care Environment has also been published as *The Hospice Journal*, Volume 12, Number 2 1997.

Cover design by Thomas J. Mayshock Jr.

Library of Congress Cataloging-in-Publication Data

Ethics in hospice care: challenges to hospice values in a changing health care environment/Bruce Jennings, editor.
    p. cm.
    "Ethics in hospice care: challenges to hospice values in a changing health care environment" has also been published as The Hospice journal, volume 12, number 2 1997"–T.p. verso.
    Includes bibliographical references and index.
    ISBN 0-7890-0328-7 (alk. paper)
    1. Hospice care–Moral and ethical aspects. 2. Hospice care–United States. I. Jennings, Bruce, 1949. II. The Hospice journal.
R726.8.E88 1997
362.1'756'0973–dc21
                                                     97-7840
                                                     CIP

ISBN 13: 978-1-138-96901-8 (pbk)
ISBN 13: 978-0-7890-0328-7 (hbk)

Ethics in Hospice Care: Challenges to Hospice Values in a Changing Health Care Environment

CONTENTS

ABOUT THE EDITOR

Bruce Jennings, MA, is Executive Vice President of The Hastings Center, a prominent research and educational institute that studies ethical and social issues in medicine, the life sciences, and the professions, and Lecturer at the Yale University School of Public Health. He has been a consultant to several governmental and private organizations, including the American Hospital Association, the W.K. Kellogg Foundation, and the March of Dimes Birth Defects Foundation. Mr. Jennings also serves on the board of directors of several national organizations, including American Health Decisions, the American Association of Bioethics, and the New York State Hospice Association. He has written and edited 13 books and has published numerous articles on bioethics and public policy issues.

Foreword

My initial contact with hospice was offering to sponsor what turned out to be the first hospice licensing law in any state when I was a member of the Florida State Senate. That was in 1979. Ten years later, the hospice founder who was the strongest advocate for the legislation, Rev. Hugh Westbrook, asked me to head the Hospice Foundation of America, which he and his wife had started in conjunction with their hospice.

The foundation's policy is to bring together persons with expertise in particular issues, discuss them thoroughly, and then arrange to have the findings published and disseminated. In 1995-96 the Hospice Foundation of America has supported The Hastings Center in conducting a study of ethical and policy issues in hospice.

The papers collected here are the product of this project. The various articles address the very real problems facing hospices in the swiftly changing health care world. Readers will be able to observe how hospices are dealing with the myriad ethical issues which are a natural result of taking care of dying people and their families. Between the lines of these papers lurks what I consider to be a major phenomenon, the rapid and unplanned growth of the hospice movement.

From a single hospice in 1973 to over 2,500 today is an incredible outburst of spontaneous compassion. I think this is partly a rejection of over-technologized medicine, partly a reaction against the dehumanization of the medical profession due to over-specialization and over commercialization, and partly a real desire on the part of many to be involved in caring for others on a personal level. It is this human dimension that attracts all of us, and which we hope will be better understood by readers of this volume.

Jack D. Gordon
President
The Hospice Foundation of America

[Haworth co-indexing entry note]: "Foreword." Gordon, Jack D. Co-published simultaneously in *The Hospice Journal* (The Haworth Press, Inc.) Vol. 12, No. 2, 1997, p. xv; and: *Ethics in Hospice Care: Challenges to Hospice Values in a Changing Health Care Environment* (ed: Bruce Jennings) The Haworth Press, Inc., 1997, p. xiii. Single or multiple copies of this article are available for a fee from The Haworth Document Delivery Service [1-800-342-9678, 9:00 a.m. - 5:00 p.m. (EST). E-mail address: getinfo@haworth.com].

Preface

In 1994, The Hastings Center began a two year research and educational project on Ethical and Policy Issues in Hospice Care, with support from
the Hospice Foundation of America. The project was stimulated by our
perception that the hospice movement and hospice organizations are facing new kinds of pressures and challenges in the 1990s; challenges that
call for closer attention to the value dimensions of hospice care. The aim
of the project is to produce new studies and educational materials on
hospice ethics that would be useful to professionals in the field.

Among these challenges are financial pressures as policy makers limit
Medicare spending; organizational pressures as hospice organizations enter a variety of new relationships with managed care organizations, home
health agencies, and hospitals; and, finally, cultural and social challenges
as Americans wrestle with moral and legal issues of death and dying,
physician-assisted suicide, and the like.

Moreover, hospice services only reach a fraction of the patients and
families who could benefit from them. Patients with end-stage AIDS or
Alzheimer's disease, terminally ill children, nursing home residents, and
various ethnic communities all continue to present hospice with the challenge of meeting their special needs.

The papers presented here were originally commissioned for The Hastings Center project on Ethical and Policy Issues in Hospice Care. Their
aim is to address the economic, social, and cultural challenges facing
hospice care today and to contribute to what must be an ongoing discussion of ethical issues and values in this vital and most humane part of our
health care system.

I would like to acknowledge the assistance and support of Jack Gordon
and the Hospice Foundation of America. Each of the papers presented here

[Haworth co-indexing entry note]: "Preface." Jennings, Bruce. Co-published simultaneously in *The Hospice Journal* (The Haworth Press, Inc.) Vol. 12, No. 2, 1997, pp. xvii-xviii; and: *Ethics in Hospice Care: Challenges to Hospice Values in a Changing Health Care Environment* (ed: Bruce Jennings) The Haworth Press, Inc., 1997, pp. xv-xvi. Single or multiple copies of this article are available for a fee from The Haworth Document Delivery Service [1-800-342-9678, 9:00 a.m. - 5:00 p.m. (EST). E-mail address: getinfo@haworth.com].

xv

benefited from the deliberations of The Hastings Center hospice ethics research group, and sincere thanks are due to the following individuals who, together with the authors of the papers collected here, served as members of that group: Philip Boyle, Richard Brett, Thomas Bryant, Daniel Callahan, Christine Cassel, Charles Corr, Randall DuFour, Joseph Fins, Kathleen Foley, Marianne Gillan, Beatrice Greenbaum, David Joranson, Grace Lee, Joanne Lynn, Ellen McGee, Ellen Moskowitz, Hilde Nelson, James Nelson, Laurence O'Connell, Ginette Olsen, Melanie Pratt, Mildred Solomon, Amy Stern, Bill Wallace, and Jane Weber.

Finally I would like to thank my colleagues on the staff of The Hastings Center who assisted with the preparation of this collection: Leigh Turner, Jennifer Stuber, Mary Ann Hasbrouck, and Marion Leyds.

Bruce Jennings
The Hastings Center

Individual Rights and the Human Good
in Hospice

Bruce Jennings

SUMMARY. Hospice care today faces economic, cultural, and so-cial challenges that will force it to rethink its basic ethical mission and its basic values if it is to grow and prosper. Three different val-ues can be said to inspire the hospice movement: palliation and the relief of suffering, enhancing individual control and autonomy at the end of life, and the value of healing or maintaining meaning and per-sonal integrity in the dying process. An emphasis on palliation alone will not be sufficient to sustain a comprehensive hospice benefit in the future. An emphasis on patient autonomy alone is not in keeping with the history or spirit of the hospice movement, which in fact has had a vision of "good" dying. The notion of healing or making whole provides the richest and most adequate concept upon which to ground the social and ethical case for hospice care in the future. *[Article copies available for a fee from The Haworth Document Delivery Service: 1-800-342-9678. E-mail address: getinfo@haworth.com]*

Hospice care represents a distinctive approach to the needs of terminally ill patients and their families. Hospice reflects its own systematic set of values and offers a vital alternative to invasive and aggressive modes of treatment found elsewhere in the health care system. While the hospice

Bruce Jennings, MA, is Executive Vice President of The Hastings Center. He is also a member of the Board of the New York State Hospice Association.

Address correspondence to: Bruce Jennings, The Hastings Center, 255 Elm Road, Briarcliff Manor, NY 10510.

[Haworth co-indexing entry note]: "Individual Rights and the Human Good in Hospice." Jennings, Bruce. Co-published simultaneously in *The Hospice Journal* (The Haworth Press, Inc.) Vol. 12, No. 2, 1997, pp. 1-7; and: *Ethics in Hospice Care: Challenges to Hospice Values in a Changing Health Care Environment* (ed: Bruce Jennings) The Haworth Press, Inc., 1997, pp. 1-7. Single or multiple copies of this article are available for a fee from The Haworth Document Delivery Service [1-800-342-9678, 9:00 a.m. - 5:00 p.m. (EST). E-mail address: getinfo@haworth.com].

1

alternative is becoming more well known and more widely utilized than ever before, its traditional values and mission are in need of continuing clarification and examination.

Hospice care professionals–including physicians, nurses, social workers, health aides, and other allied health professionals–frequently confront ethical dilemmas in practice. How well are these dilemmas understood? How cogently and openly are they discussed?

THE CHALLENGE OF CHANGE

At one level, hospice is one of the most self-consciously "moral" and "ethical" sectors of the entire health care system. Its origins lie in a social and ethical movement, and an ethic of compassion, dignity, and service. Paradoxically, however, perhaps due to this value-based heritage, systematic reflection on ethics in the hospice field is curiously underdeveloped. In the past the value commitments of hospice may have been seen as self-evident, noncontroversial, and in need of little explicit analysis and examination.

If that assumption was ever true (which I doubt), it is certainly no longer true today. In the 1990s the hospice philosophy of care is undergoing change and challenge, as are hospices as organizations. In part this is due to structural and economic transformations in the health care system as a whole, and to the current uncertainty about the direction of health policy reform. In a time of government Medicare cutbacks and cost-containment under the increasing supervision of managed care systems in the private sector, will already financially frugal hospice services be able to maintain an adequate level and quality of care? As priorities in health policy shift toward primary and preventive care, will the palliative care and psycho-social support of dying patients and their families receive their fair share of resources?

This time of debate and ferment in the hospice community is also a reflection of the cultural and value changes taking place in American society, particularly on issues of death and dying. The U.S. Supreme Count decision in the *Cruzan* case was a capstone to several years of court affirmation at the state level of the patient's right to forgo life-sustaining treatment, a viewpoint the hospice movement heralded long before it was fashionable or politically popular. Now, however, many in society seem ready to move further and to embrace physician assisted suicide and voluntary, active euthanasia. Today, central tenets such as death with dignity, natural dying, the prevention and relief of suffering, and the like cannot be left unanalyzed or taken for granted.

Hospice professionals will benefit from a broader and deeper dialogue on ethical issues and from continuing education and in-service training programs on bioethics to enhance decisionmaking in their own practice. Hospice administration faces financial and regulatory issues that raise ethical dilemmas both for individual care givers and for hospices as organizations. These issues also need to be confronted forthrightly, with clear reasoning and sound ethical principles in view.

THREE FACES OF HOSPICE

As an outside observer of the field, it is my impression that there are basically three ways in which most people conceive of the core mission of hospice. There are three moral faces of hospice.

Palliation. The first of these is that hospice is about relief of pain and suffering when one's terminal illness (usually cancer) has progressed to the point where it is "hopeless," and "nothing more is to be done." Hospitals can't do much for you any more, and it's best if possible to go home to be near your family when you die. Doctors who aim for cure have done with you and pass you along to other doctors and nurses who specialize in making the best of a losing situation. In this conception, hospice essentially promises patients: "We will stand by you so you will not die in unbearable pain, and you will not die alone." There are many misconceptions and very destructive assumptions built into this notion of hospice—particularly the negative image of hospice as a dumping ground, a faute de mieux—and some kernels of moral truth as well, such as the element of witness and commitment. But for good or ill, it has been a tenacious image in the public mind, and hospice hasn't yet shaken it.

Autonomy. The second conception of hospice I observe focuses less on relief of pain and suffering than on respect for the rights and autonomy of the dying person. In this emphasis, hospice certainly shares a core value now influential throughout the entire health care system, but it also smacks of the particular heritage of hospice as a grassroots, alternative care movement. To many, acute care medicine at the end of life, with its ICUs, its invasive life-support technologies, its "heroic" and experimental oncology treatments, is a very negative symbol of loss of personal dignity and control. Hospice is a haven of autonomy in a high tech medical world. Long before the courts had finally settled the issue in a remarkably convoluted series of appellate level court decisions from the *Quinlan* case in 1976 to the *Cruzan* case in 1989, hospice had affirmed the right of the competent patient to refuse life-sustaining medical treatment as a philosophical and an ethical matter. Hospice can't keep a person from dying, but it can preserve and respect the values of the dying person in the dying process. Autonomy means the freedom or the right to live your own life your own way, so long as you don't harm or violate the rights of others. Autonomy in hospice means the right to die your own death in your own way.

Healing. Finally, there is an understanding of hospice that stresses neither palliation, nor autonomy, but some substantive conception of "good dying," or more accurately, "the good in dying." This notion is harder to pin down, but I believe that it has been and remains influential. Its core idea is captured in the slogan that hospice is not about death, it's about living up to the time of death. The ending chapter of one's life, whether it be a few months, weeks, or days, is as important as any other chapter in the biography of a person. Life, even in this last chapter, has its own capacity for flourishing, its own integrity and intrinsic worth. What is required for this final flourishing are human goods that go beyond freedom from pain and freedom from outside interference; as necessary as the goods of palliation and autonomy are, they are not sufficient to create a good living near death, they are not sufficient to promote the human good at the end of life. Since the mission of hospice, according to this view, is to promote the human good at the end of life, the ethics of hospice must look beyond palliation and autonomy. What it seeks is threefold: (1) sustaining relationships, (2) sustaining the integrity of the self, and (3) achieving an appropriate closure to one's life through reconciliation with one's past, one's self-identity, and with others. These three goals can be summed up in a single word: healing. The root meaning of healing is "making whole." The mission of hospice is to facilitate healing in this sense.

THE PLACE OF THE GOOD IN HOSPICE ETHICS

Having set out these three different conceptions of the goal of hospice care, my thesis is that the third notion is much more important than the first two, and, I think, more philosophically defensible. But the strengths and weaknesses of this hospice vision of the human good at the end of life, relative to the ethics of compassion and palliation and the ethic of autonomy, have not yet been assessed adequately. Doing so should be high on the agenda of future discussions of hospice ethics.

I will be reminded that the three distinctions just drawn are artificial and that these values actually blend into one another in real life and practice; and so they do. But the function of these artificial and analytic distinctions is to clarify and refine ideas, not to describe actual practice, which will always be a mix and blending of many values. To sharpen the distinction between promoting autonomy and promoting a substantive understanding of the human good at the end of life is the first step toward a more in-depth treatment of ethical issues in hospice.

One of the most interesting aspects of hospice is that it is at once very individually oriented, and at the same time it is inevitably involved in an enterprise of reshaping the patient's relationship with others, particularly family members. Perhaps it is better to say that the illness is reshaping those relationships, but hospice at least has to accommodate everyone involved to that harsh reality. For good therapeutic as well as ethical reasons, hospice must be individually oriented because the patient must be treated as a subject, an active participant and partner in the process of his or her own care. In hospice, therefore, the notion of respect for patient autonomy is central. But it has a different meaning than it often does in acute care settings, because in hospice to respect autonomy does not mean giving the patient anything like the normal scope of life choices and abilities which permit autonomy to be exercised. To advocate for autonomy and rights alone in the hospice context is to abstract from the reality of the patient's medical and psychological situation. If the concept of autonomy is to function as a moral compass for care givers in hospice, it must somehow be linked with notions of dependency and relationship much more so that it normally has been in broader discussions of medical ethics and law.

Someone, like myself, who wants to affirm that the goals and relationships arising in hospice are linked more to a substantive conception of the good (captured in the concept of "healing") than to autonomy and rights, faces a steep uphill climb in a pluralistic and secular society. This is because in American society an important ethical tenet of individual freedom says that no conception of the good should be imposed on a person by others. As individuals in a pluralistic social order, we are self-defining, and the freedom to define ourselves and our own good in our own way is an essential part of the good life itself.

How are we to capture the significance of *relationships* in hospice care in this individualistic climate? Doesn't it seem stilted and abstract to speak of the isolated individual patient making choices and directing professional care-givers in a contractual transaction governed by patient preferences? In fact, isn't it most often closer to the mark to say that the "choices" and decisions tend to emerge out of ongoing interactions among patient, family, and the hospice team? Medical choices are rarely made by the atomistic individuals of liberal social theory, least of all in hospice.

This analysis suggests that a central ethical challenge of the care giver-patient relationship in hospice is to overcome the following dilemma: Every moral instinct in our liberal, pluralistic society tells us that all competent adults should be able to define their own good in their own way. At the same time, both the medical and social realities of terminal illness belie this atomistic picture of individual self-fashioning and self-sovereignty. Meaning comes through relationships, empowerment through dependency, and the goal is not to shape circumstances but to be shaped by unchosen circumstances in the most affirming way feasible. Only through therapeutic and caregiving relationships of a special type can the patient's good be mutually discovered rather than unilaterally imposed by another. Only in that way can one walk the line between a demeaning and manipulative professional paternalism, on the one hand, and a kind of formal respect for autonomy that is inattentive to the human reality of dying, on the other.

From what source will hospice draw a moral vocabulary rich enough to articulate the profession's proper sense of social and ethical purpose? Where is the vocabulary needed to express why society ought to value the caring and the healing hospice can provide, why scarce resources ought to be devoted to it, and why society should make an investment in hospice adequate to allow it to nurture with adequate facilities and resources the fragile and morally complex relationships that do (and should) evolve between providers and patients at the end of life?

Unfortunately, there is a large gap between the vocabulary that bioethics–and the underlying social ethos of a liberal individualistic culture– gives us to discuss the goals and relationships of hospice care, and the lived experience and reality of that care. If this gap grows too large, it becomes dangerous because individual professionals and ordinary patients alike will become alienated from the discussions of ethics that occur at more elite, policy-making and regulatory levels. Ethics must speak directly to the constraints and realities we face. Unrealistic and inappropriate notions of autonomy, independence, and the like produce conflict and frustration rather than empowerment and respect.

The gap between the moral vocabulary of autonomy and the lived realities for hospice professionals, patients, and families is also dangerous in a time of cost-containment and priority-setting in the broader health care system. Increasingly, hospice will have to justify the social expenditures made on its behalf. The terms in which this social justification will be made are not yet clear. Certain narrow conceptions of technology assessment, and equally narrow conceptions of quality of life, have a great deal of influence in policy circles today. In my opinion, they threaten to underestimate and to undervalue precisely those aspects of care and healing within dependence and limitation that are among hospice's greatest strengths.

To make the social case for support for hospice in the future will require finding the right moral vocabulary for appraising the good that hospice serves. The wisdom of hospice reminds us that all individuals will die, and that until then we all live and flourish in and through relationships of mutual giving and interdependency. To live well, or perhaps more precisely, to live the human good; to be healed, and to be sustained meaningfully whole–these things are to grow, to change, to be transformed. These are the goods of hospice because they are as much a part of the human life story in its final pages as they are at the beginning of the book.

Issues of Access in a Diverse Society

Paul R. Brenner

SUMMARY. Hospices are successful in addressing the needs of middle class, white, elderly persons with cancer who have family members able to care for them at home. However, there is a need to provide better access to care within diverse settings and for diverse populations. Ethnic minorities, marginalized persons and those without stable home environments or living in nontraditional ways are not well served by hospice at the present time. To improve access to hospice care, hospices need to address the distinctive profiles of their staffs and make them more inclusive and representative of the total community for their service area, create a broad range of programs of outreach, build bridges with other programs, develop expanded resources to manage the needs of patients and families, and train volunteers and staff to work in non-traditional home settings. *[Article copies available from The Haworth Document Delivery Service: 1-800-342-9678. E-mail address: getinfo@haworth.com]*

Influenced by the early work of Elisabeth Kubler-Ross in the United States, and borrowing from the work of Dame Cicely Saunders at St. Christopher's Hospice, London during the 1960s, the hospice movement in the United States in the 1970s had a vision of what constituted a "good death":

Paul R. Brenner is Executive Director, Jacob Perlow Hospice, Beth Israel Health Care System, New York City. He also serves as Chairman of the Board of the New York State Hospice Association and is a member of the AIDS Resource Committee of the National Hospice Organization.

Address correspondence to: Paul R. Brenner, Jacob Perlow Hospice, First Avenue at 16th Street, New York, NY 10003.

[Haworth co-indexing entry note]: "Issues of Access in a Diverse Society." Brenner, Paul R. Co-published simultaneously in *The Hospice Journal* (The Haworth Press, Inc.) Vol. 12, No. 2, 1997, pp. 9-16; and: *Ethics in Hospice Care: Challenges to Hospice Values in a Changing Health Care Environment* (ed: Bruce Jennings) The Haworth Press, Inc., 1997, pp. 9-16. Single or multiple copies of this article are available for a fee from The Haworth Document Delivery Service [1-800-342-9678, 9:00 a.m. - 5:00 p.m. (EST). E-mail address: getinfo@haworth.com].

- At home, not in a hospital.
- Surrounded by family, not alone.
- Comfortable, not in uncontrolled pain.
- Peaceful, not struggling with fear, denial, anger and bargaining.

The first American hospice began service in 1974. Funded through a founding grant which limited care to patients with cancer, it provided the basic model around which other hospices were organized throughout the 1970s. At the end of the 1970s the Health Care Financing Administration (HCFA) established a Hospice Demonstration Project with a select number of developing hospices. On the basis of that information, Congress added hospices to the Medicare program at the beginning of Ronald Reagan's first term as president.

The Medicare hospice benefit was the first comprehensive reimbursement mechanism created for hospice services. Its conditions of participation became a national standard to define hospice care as well. Since 1983, there has been a rapid increase in the number of hospice providers and patients served. By the end of 1995, there were approximately 1,800 Medicare certified hospices in the United States.

ASSUMPTIONS

The structure of the Medicare benefit is based on some fundamental assumptions from the experience of the hospices of the 1970s. Among these, four are most significant.

1. *Informed Consent.* Hospice is understood as a choice a patient makes for a certain kind of treatment philosophy and set of services.
2. *Alternative Care.* Hospice is understood as a different option for care at the ending of life in contrast to a curative acute care focused model.
3. *Presence of Definable Progressive Terminal Illness.* Hospice is understood as being available to patients for whom a terminal prognosis of six months or less can be determined by a licensed physician.
4. *Home Care.* Hospice is understood as providing a different setting for care in the following ways: first, the predominant place of care is the patient's own home. Second, the predominant source of care is the patient's own family. Third, the predominant kind of care provided by hospice is intermittent skilled and supportive care to supplement the family's own care, not replace it. Finally, inpatient care is provided only as support for brief episodes of need that cannot be provided in the home, not as a basic placement for care.

CURRENT STATUS AND FUTURE CHALLENGES

According to recent information available from the National Hospice Organization (Hospice Fact Sheet, October 10, 1995), the following characterizes hospice activity:

- 37% of all who died of cancer related causes in the United States were cared for by hospices.
- 78% of all care provided by all hospice programs was provided to persons with cancer.
- 31% of all who died of AIDS-related causes received hospice services.
- AIDS care represented 4% of the total cases cared for by hospices.
- Hospices served a patient base that was 85% white, 15% non-white.
- Hospices were staffed by personnel who were 90% white, 10% non-white.
- 65% of all patients served were covered by Medicare.
- 7% of all patients served were covered by Medicaid.
- 70% of all patients were 65 years or older.

When these statistics are set against the original mission of serving the terminally ill and the families, it is clear that hospice has been relatively successful in serving middle class elderly white persons with cancer who have family members available and willing to care for them at home.

It is also clear that hospices as a whole have not been successful in providing access to care to persons and illnesses which diverge from this basic profile.

Examples of patients who have been challenging for hospices to reach and serve include those with basic living needs deficits, such as:

- Those who live alone and/or are socially isolated.
- Those who have severely malfunctioning and conflicted families.
- Those who live in unsafe or remote areas where hospice care givers are reluctant or unable to go.
- Those who do not have a stable or safe living environment at home.
- Those who do have consistent basic necessities, such as utilities, phone, food, hot running water, heat, or income.
- Those who are homeless, live in shelters, SROs, or in other non-traditional housing situations.

The family and home settings of these kinds of patients do not easily facilitate the implementation of hospice care, which depends upon basic primary care already being in place and being provided by family members in a secure, comfortable environment.

The ways in which individuals gain access to medical care also affects how difficult it may be for hospice programs to serve them. Such considerations include:

- Those who use the Medicaid system to meet their health needs.
- Those who have no third party payer source or financial resources to self-pay for services.
- Those who use emergency systems as the primary care physician.
- Those who are in the care of public health clinics, or other similar systems such as for Native Americans, or persons who are incarcerated.

Most hospice programs require patients to have a consistent primary attending physician with whom the hospice team coordinates care. The absence of such a physician can also block access to care.

Moreover, there are individuals who live outside the traditional dominant culture and/or its institutions. These persons comprise various stigmatized, displaced, and/or disenfranchised populations, such as:

- Gay men and lesbian women.
- Adults and children of color, African, Asian, Caribbean, Hispanic.
- Persons whose primary language is not English.
- The institutionalized mentally ill.
- Persons with addictions to drugs or alcohol.
- Prisoners.
- Refugees, immigrants, illegal residents.
- Migrant workers and their families.
- Native Americans and others whose culture is non-European-based and oriented.

Related to these issues are the complex ways cultural, social, class and racial factors influence access to care and the ability of hospices to implement services. Many of these factors originate in fundamental differences between basic assumptions of hospice staff and volunteers and those of the patients and families being served. The following identifies some of these significant differences.

What is meant by the word family? Who is automatically included and excluded? What makes a person a part of a family? Is the family patriarchal of matriarchal in its organization? Who is the head both functionally and structurally? What is the role and status of the elders? How is communication managed within the family and what are the structures through which it flows? How are children included in its life?

What is the role of religion? How do beliefs influence what choices are possible? What practices are considered necessary? Where does religious authority reside? What is the relationship with the religious leader, whether priest, minister, rabbi, holy person, or shaman? How is conflict between religious ideals or mandates and the actual condition or situation handled? What are the inter-connections between religion, culture, ethnicity, language, and class?

What are understood as basic roles assigned to each gender? What are men supposed to be like and do? What are women supposed to be like and do? How do the genders relate? How are caregiving activities and roles linked to gender? What expectations do family members and patients have of professional staff members and volunteers that are influenced by gender assumptions? How are masculine and feminine values and characteristics linked to gender and institutionalized in the culture? How does religion play a role in this genderization?

What are the understandings of sexuality in the patient's and family's cultural values and practice? How is sexual deviance regarded and discussed? Is one's sexuality determined by the gender of the person one is intimate with or the role one plays regardless of the gender of the other? What are the operating prohibitions and permissions that affect discussion of sexual behavior and identity? How do the practices and beliefs of religion affect the practice of sexuality?

What are the boundaries of individual choice and autonomy? Is the individual the highest value, or the family, or the group? How are decisions made and who is involved in the decision-making process? Is choice and decision making based on a participatory, inclusionary process or a hierarchial structure?

What meanings and values are ascribed to words like "health," "well-being," "quality of life," "disease," "healing"? What are indigenous beliefs and practices for managing illness and health? Who are its practitioners? What does the patient and family understand about the medical system and its institutions, and what kind of relationship with it do they have? What understandings does the patient have about his or her medical condition?

What is truth telling? What kind of information can and cannot be shared? What are the ways in which truth can be shared? What kinds of truth can be discussed comfortably and what kinds cannot be? What conflicts are there between expectations regarding truth telling?

What is the relationship of the group to which the patient and family are members and outsiders who are members of the dominant society? What are the rules governing the behavior and role of outsiders? How does an outsider establish credibility, demonstrate appropriate behavior and vocabulary, and offer services? How does the patient and family interpret their place within this relationship and the experience of their group's history with the dominant culture, its institutions and its representatives?

How are dying and death understood? What practices are a part of dying and death? How are dying and death discussed? Who is appropriate to involve in these discussions and who is not? Is there a proper or desirable place in which death is expected to occur? Are there special considerations involved in arranging for death to occur at home?

What are the rituals, practices, beliefs and values surrounding the expression and understanding of loss, mourning, grief, and bereavement? What are considered to be appropriate ways to express and discuss them?

In addition to all these considerations, a significant factor of access also involves the age of the patient, especially if he or she is a dependent minor child. The illnesses, congenital conditions, and medical conditions which affect children and how they are managed is very different from an "end stage/terminal" management model for adults. There are profound developmental considerations which influence the practice of consent and choice, and necessitate work with parents and/or legal guardians. In the more recent expansion of AIDS to children, all the additional complications of that disease are imposed as well upon already difficult issues for children, especially because a number of these children are from lower-income families of color, have infected and sick parents, and confront hospice programs with issues involving child placement, foster care, and adoption. Sometimes these children are being raised by grandparents because the birth-parents have already died.

Finally, there is a cluster of problems for hospices relating to medical conditions which do not follow the definable progressive terminal model of cancer or have other complicating factors. These include:

- Diseases that primarily affect marginalized and/or stigmatized populations.
- Illnesses that are long term chronic conditions.
- Diseases which affect the mental capacities of patients to make treatment decisions or participate in care.
- Diseases for which there is no cure but are treated aggressively with life-extending procedures and/or drugs.
- Diseases which are complicated by other diagnoses, such as mental illness or addictions, or other medical conditions, such as ventilators or dialysis.
- Diseases that have a different kind of trajectory, such as childhood conditions, AIDS, or ALS.

What is the role of hospice care with persons whose care needs for end-of-life support may not fall within a six month criteria standard?

- How does one determine what is "end stage" in diseases that are not "progressively terminal" in a way similar to that of cancer?
- What is the role of hospice with persons who are ventilator dependent or on dialysis?
- What is the role of hospice care with patients who are cognitively impaired or unresponsive?
- How early is it appropriate for hospice to intervene and become involved with patients and families?

These differing kinds of medical conditions create challenging issues for hospices.

RECOMMENDATIONS

There is a critical interdependence, interrelationship and intersection of factors which may block the ability of individuals needing end-of-life care to access hospice services. Any of these factors taken alone or together may challenge the historic ways hospices have offered their services, understood their role, and achieved value for their work. Therefore, the following issues identify an agenda for hospice programs to examine in order to expand access of care to individuals and families who are not primarily a part of the dominant society and its values.

1. Hospices must address the racial-cultural-ethnic-language-class-gender-age profile of their professional and volunteer staffs and governing bodies in order to make them more inclusive and representative of the total community of their service area.
2. Hospices must create a broad range of programs of outreach to build relationships with the communities which have largely not accessed hospice services.
3. Hospices must build bridges with other programs, services and institutions in their communities which provide care for the disenfranchised, economically deprived and disadvantaged members of various minority communities, and others outside the dominant culture in order to develop the cultural competence of their programs and staffs and provide access to care.
4. Hospices must develop expanded resources to manage the needs of patients and families that fall outside the range of reimbursed ser-

vices, such as primary care, basic living necessities, including housing, and other special needs.
5. Hospices must train their staffs and volunteers to work effectively
and comfortably in a wide range of non-traditional home settings,
neighborhoods, institutions, as well as remote areas.
6. Hospices must see themselves not as an isolated self-contained service delivery system but as an integral part of the health care continuum and a full participant in the social contract and its structures and
values.
7. Hospices must see their expanding social and cultural role in their
communities as an extension of their creative tradition and history.

The ability of the hospice movement to address these issues successfully
will move it from a system which serves a select population which is
easiest to serve, to a system which influences the way all dying persons in
America receive care at life's ending.

Will Assisted Suicide Kill Hospice?

Arthur L. Caplan

SUMMARY. Hospice is often held out as an alternative to the need for assisted suicide. To date, those in the hospice movement have made any discussion of assistance in dying off-limits on the grounds that proper palliative care can address the concerns about pain that the terminally ill face.

But, the movement toward assisted suicide raises questions about the future viability of the hospice movement in its current form. Many who see assistance in dying are concerned, not about pain, but about suffering and loss of dignity. Many are not terminally ill but terrified at the prospect of disability and loss of cognitive capacities. Unless hospice addresses these concerns it is not likely to survive in the face of pressures to legalize assisted suicide. *[Article copies available from The Haworth Document Delivery Service: 1-800-342-9678. E-mail address: getinfo@haworth.com]*

The hospice movement in America is in big trouble. It stands a good chance of becoming the first victim of the burgeoning movement to legalize assisted suicide. The pressures to rein in the escalating costs of health care, a chronic care system that is often more a source of fear than comfort, and an inadequate appreciation on the part of the public and legislators of what hospice does may all combine to condemn this important form of care to a tragic, premature death.

Arthur L. Caplan, PhD, is Director of the Center for Bioethics and Trustee Professor at the University of Pennsylvania.

Address correspondence to: Arthur L. Caplan, Center for Bioethics, University of Pennsylvania, 3401 Market Street, Philadelphia, PA 19104.

[Haworth co-indexing entry note]: "Will Assisted Suicide Kill Hospice?" Caplan, Arthur L. Co-published simultaneously in *The Hospice Journal* (The Haworth Press, Inc.) Vol. 12, No. 2, 1997, pp. 17-24; and: *Ethics in Hospice Care: Challenges to Hospice Values in a Changing Health Care Environment* (ed: Bruce Jennings) The Haworth Press, Inc., 1997, pp. 17-24. Single or multiple copies of this article are available for a fee from The Haworth Document Delivery Service [1-800-342-9678, 9:00 a.m. - 5:00 p.m. (EST). E-mail address: getinfo@haworth.com].

CAN HOSPICE SURVIVE THE LEGALIZATION OF ASSISTED SUICIDE?

For decades the moral ideology behind hospice has been grounded in patient choice, self-determination, and the importance of maintaining the quality of life even during the process of dying. Hospice is offered to some who are dying–primarily adults with disseminated cancer–as an alternative to efforts at long-shot intensive efforts to extend life. For many, hospice seems a far better choice than dying intubated, monitored, poked, prodded, undermedicated, and aggressively resuscitated by strangers in an unfamiliar and uncomfortable environment. The rationale for hospice is closely linked to the reality facing those with very advanced forms of cancer and other terminal illnesses. The terminally ill are almost always better off (from their own point of view and that of their family and friends) with care, attentiveness, spiritual support, and conversation rather than undergoing Herculean efforts to secure additional hours or days of life of exceedingly poor quality.

An essential element for the functioning of hospice is trust. There must be trust between the patient and the care provider, between the patient and the hospice organization, and between the care provider and the patient's family or significant others. Without trust, those seeking hospice services could not be sure that they had really pursued all reasonable courses of medical intervention to extend their lives. They could not be sure that they had not been sent to hospice to die cheaply rather than to die well. Without trust, the ministrations that are the core of hospice care are neither credible nor effective, as recent work on the importance of trust to therapeutic efficacy suggests. Without trust, some patients and their families would wonder whether the actions taken by hospice workers were always in the best interest of the patient.

Prior to the emergence of the movement to legitimize assisted suicide and euthanasia, those in hospice care could place complete trust in their hospice care providers. There was almost no reason to fear that anyone had been placed in hospice prematurely, that someone would be sent to a hospice if there were still potentially efficacious therapies to be tried, nor that those providing care would not do everything in their power to extend life while maintaining the dignity and quality of that life. The ethos of hospice was that hastening death, hurrying death, or assisting in death had no place in hospice treatment. This was clear and comforting.

Events have changed. One state, Oregon, has enacted a law allowing assisted suicide, and other states may follow suit. Some high Federal courts believe a right to assistance in dying can be found in the constitution. Doctors and nurses indicate that they will and should sometimes intentionally bring about the death of a patient, sometimes without the consent of the patient. Also we have recently witnessed the bizarre vindication and quasi-martyrdom of Dr. Jack Kevorkian. Hospice's historic abhorrence for suicide is not tenable. The negative liberty to refuse medical treatment is rapidly being joined with the positive right to an entitlement to help in dying in American law. The winds of autonomy are blowing death away from hospice toward a very different location.

Agree or not, like it or not, these shifts in public policy have cast a pall over the historical ethos of hospice and thus over the requisite trust. When hastening death becomes an option, the trust necessary to make hospice function as a place where dying is an unhurried, humane affair is in jeopardy.

WHY THE NEED FOR ASSISTANCE IN DYING?

The debate about assisted suicide is always cast in terms of personal self-determination, but it actually has less to do with this value than might be supposed. Individuals have always had the right to end their lives regardless of what others may think of the morality of such an action and only a tiny handful of the terminally ill are so frail and incompetent that they cannot do so if they so choose. The struggle to legalize assisted suicide is really about a number of other matters: fear, guilt, cost and dignity. Hospice emerged as one way to respond to these concerns. Assisted suicide is now emerging as another. The two are unlikely to coexist for very long.

Fear, not self-determination, is fueling the push toward making assisted suicide by doctors legal. Many people are afraid of being kept alive under circumstances they abhor, but they are also afraid they will lack the means, the knowledge or even the courage to kill themselves. They want competent help available to them when they die, not because they lack the ability to act freely and autonomously to kill themselves, but because they fear they will lack the willpower to do what they want to do when the time to do it comes.

When fear is mixed with guilt an especially potent brew is created, one strong enough to undercut support for hospice and to bring assisted suicide to the forefront of public policy. In many circles it is still seen as immoral or sinful to take your own life. Suicide may not be illegal but many believe it to be immoral. Some are not so sure but do not want to take a chance in the hereafter about the morality of suicide.

Assistance in dying relieves the individual of carrying the personal moral burden for ending one's own life. It also spares having to ask family or friends to carry this responsibility. In a society that is eager to assign responsibility for many unpleasant or uncomfortable things to others, especially to professionals, assisted suicide looks like a far more attractive option than taking personal responsibility for the decision to end one's life and then acting upon it.

Cost is also fueling the effort to change the law to allow assistance in dying by doctors. Money is not a welcome visitor at debates about assisted suicide, but it is present nonetheless. Many Americans do not want to spend their resources on the final weeks and days of their dying. Still others believe that it is irresponsible to family and even to society to linger around, consuming resources once death is inevitable. Still others believe that the only way this nation is going to solve the fiscal burden of an aging society is to find ways to spend less money at the end of life. While not always bluntly articulated when the discussion turns to care for the dying, these views are omnipresent whenever economists and public officials talk behind closed doors. The desire to save money creates an atmosphere in which assisted suicide by physicians looks very attractive, surely more attractive than spending the money it would take to upgrade a flagging long-term and chronic care system, and perhaps even more attractive than the smaller amounts of money it would take to provide good quality hospice services to all who might benefit.

Quality of life, as distinct from the quality of one's dying, is also a key ingredient in the assisted suicide debate. Much has been made in the debate over assisted suicide of the importance of controlling pain. And it is true that too many Americans die in pain. However, pain is not the issue fueling public support for assisted suicide. What most Americans fear is the loss of the capacity to think and feel, to ambulate and emote, to control their bowels and bladder. Most people understand that there is every reason to believe that they can be kept comfortable and pain free if they receive even minimally competent medical treatment while dying, but that is not enough.

Severe disability, loss of cognitive function, loss of self-esteem, frailness and dependency are what people have in mind avoiding if they can choose physician assisted suicide. Hospice does nothing to answer these quality of life concerns since they have little to do with pain and terminal illness. Assisted suicide has everything to do with them.

HOSPICE DEALS WITH PAIN
BUT FOR MANY SUFFERING IS THE ISSUE

Arguments about assisted suicide, especially in the context of hospice as an alternative, often pivot around the issue of how well pain can be controlled in someone with cancer or AIDS. In fact, there is nothing to debate. Medicine and nursing know full well how to control most forms of pain. They may fail to do so but the failure has nothing to do with a lack of general knowledge about pain control. It has to do with inadequate training, callous indifference to patient requests for relief, and culpable stupidity about addiction. Even when aggressive pain relief means risking inadvertent death, most hospice workers are comfortable making pain relief a priority come what may in the form of death as a side-effect. However, pain is not the issue when it comes to assisted suicide.

The moral challenge medicine and nursing face is what to do about the management of suffering, not pain. Suffering is far broader than pain. Suffering refers to the loss of identity that occurs with a disfiguring or disabling injury. Suffering comes when you know you can no longer remember your children's names or where you live. Suffering is represented by the reality of being made a prisoner inside your own body, unable to move. A proud man or woman in a culture that makes a fetish of self-determination and independence may not be able to bear the thought of being incontinent of bowel and bladder or simply unable to answer the phone or use a toothbrush.

The answer from medicine to concerns about suffering so far has been silence. Even hospice has concentrated mainly on the management of these assaults on the self, but not on avoiding or eliminating them. Yet, for many Americans it is suffering and the erosion of self that is to be feared: this is what leads many to think about ending their lives. The concern to avoid suffering, broadly construed to include loss of dignity, self-esteem, and fear of dependency, is the strongest challenge hospice has ever faced.

FOR MANY, IMPAIRMENT IS REASON ENOUGH TO END THEIR LIVES

Most people who favor changing the law to permit assistance in dying want to place tight restrictions on who will be granted this right. In the version of the law enacted in the state of Oregon, in the decisions of Federal appellate courts and in many articles and books, it is only the terminally ill who are permitted to voluntarily elect to die with help from a doctor. One of the few who has shown no interest in restricting physician assisted suicide to terminally ill patients is Dr. Jack Kevorkian. Support for his actions has been widespread both among the public and in some quarters within the health professions despite this fact.

Kevorkian has always maintained that anyone who is competent should have the right to suicide assistance on demand. He has been willing to back this belief up with action. At least three of the persons he assisted in dying–Sherri Miller, Marjorie Wantz, and Janet Adkins–were not terminally ill.

Limiting the right to assistance in dying to those who request it makes sense. After all, no one should be helped to die against his or her will. To kill without a request is murder, not suicide. Involuntary euthanasia, at the direction of family, doctors or the state, is an especially morally suspect activity. The worst genocide in this century took place with the moral rationale that involuntary euthanasia of Jews, Gypsies, Jehovah's Witnesses, Communists, Slavs, persons with handicaps and homosexuals was ethically justified.

It is very unlikely that assistance in dying is something that will long be restricted to the terminally ill. For too many Americans, the issue of when to die involves neither terminal illness nor pain. It involves the loss of a sense of personal identity, the loss of dignity and the loss of an acceptable quality of life. This is the group that poses the greatest challenge to the tradition of hospice since many of those who fit these categories are not now and have not been candidates for eligibility for hospice, yet they are strong candidates for requesting help in dying.

Those with advanced ALS, Parkinsonism, severe arthritis, Alzheimer's, chronic severe depression, severe burns, disfiguring injuries, brain injury, advanced cystic fibrosis, massive stroke and many other disorders, diseases and impairments will press for relief from their suffering. While the hospice movement has confined its attention to those facing imminent and certain death, these groups are not concerned with such limits. Their involvement in assisted suicide threatens to overwhelm both interest in and support for hospice as a prelude to dying under any circumstances.

THE ARGUMENTS FOR ACTIVE ASSISTANCE BY HEALTH CARE PROFESSIONALS AND THEIR CONSEQUENCES FOR HOSPICE

If autonomy is placed at the center of ethical discourse in a society, as it surely is in the United States, then it is very difficult to mount a persuasive argument against the legalization of assisted suicide by health care professionals. If it is true that self-determination includes the right to decide when life has become unbearable or burdensome, and if it is also true that the only way to permit the safe and humane ending of life is through the participation of health care professionals, then the case for assisted suicide is not difficult to make on moral and political grounds.

It is a recognized fact that pain control is sometimes not what it ought to be for those who are dying and that even when pain can be controlled it sometimes requires rendering a person stuporous and incoherent, a state many find unacceptable. While those in the hospice movement may know that most cases of pain can be adequately controlled without severely impairing the cognitive capacities of the patient, it is nonetheless true that some persons will not wish to undergo a regimen of palliation while others would find their pain so severe that palliation will require a loss of mental functioning that is deemed unacceptable. Hospice has little to offer such persons.

Since no one is proposing involuntary euthanasia nor is anyone calling for the mandatory invocation of assisted suicide for those who reach a given level of impairment, proponents of changing public policy need only note that they favor the creation of the option of assisted suicide. Legalization of assisted suicide may be beneficial even for those who choose not to take this path. The mere fact that the opportunity for help in dying exists may help some persons to endure more disability or dysfunction than they otherwise might have been willing to face.

Hospice has relatively little to say in the face of such arguments. Hospice workers can say that they are morally uncomfortable with assisting in dying but such reservations do not directly meet the claim that a respect for autonomy and humaneness require making assisted suicide available if it is performed by those willing to do so. Hospice advocates may say that its treatments and techniques can give hope to many facing imminent death, but that does not address the needs of those who find what goes on in a hospice unacceptable from their own view of dignity and self-control. Those with experience in hospice can say that they have seen many patients adapt and accommodate to the realities of infirmity and incapacity which may accompany dying, but again this is not an argument that will persuade those who maintain they have a right to forego these adaptive experiences if they so wish. Unless those in hospice are prepared to radically alter the prevailing criteria for admission, there will be some patients for whom hospice cannot be an option because they are not terminally ill but who see death is desirable due to the burden of disease or impairment.

Hospice does not fare well placed against these positions. It does not meet the needs of many and for some its very mode of treatment is unacceptable. While most people, even those who are very sick, may choose to see the dying process through to the end, many will opt for assisted suicide rather than the course of palliation, support, and pain control. Eventually hospice programs will either have to incorporate assisted dying into their care plans or risk elimination by new forms of terminal illness care which include assistance in dying for those who request it.

The only way hospice in America can avoid this scenario is to try to convince Americans that a good death is not one in which a life ends abruptly, at the first sign of pain or disability. Hospice must be able not just to provide support and palliative care, but also to convince people that these are the things they need as a part of the best possible death.

Those in hospice must also be able to persuade Americans that a good death can be a relatively cheap and affordable one. Many Americans fear the economic consequences of a high technology death. They do not want to spend their resources on treatments that are perceived to be of little benefit. Similarly, if hospice care is seen as expensive or burdensome to the patient, or the patient's family, then the option of a planned death will loom as more attractive from the point of view of the bottom line, the patient's as well as society's.

I am not sure that even these steps will be sufficient to preserve the mission and philosophy of hospice as they now exist. The creation of a right to die on demand with the aid of a doctor or a nurse may simply make hospice appear to be an anachronism in the eyes of many who might once have considered it as a way to die. Hospice arose as a way to ensure a good death in a medical system overly obsessed with utilizing expensive high technology upon the dying. If it is to endure, hospice must be able to explain why the kind of death it provides is an attractive and affordable alternative to a quick, cheap and easy death at the hands of a health care professional.

Ethical Issues in Pain Management

Michael J. McCabe

SUMMARY. The modern hospice movement has played a significant role in the development of palliative care. Effective palliation is of crucial importance in achieving quality of life and a dignified death for the terminally ill. While the inherent risk in palliative care, respiratory depression, remains an open medical question, an understanding of the ethical and moral principle of double effect demonstrates the prudential nature of palliative care and how it is an application of the ethical and moral norm, respect for patient autonomy. *[Article copies available from The Haworth Document Delivery Service: 1-800-342-9678. E-mail address: getinfo@haworth.com]*

Palliative care, the hallmark of hospice care, is of crucial importance in achieving quality of life and a dignified death for the terminally ill. The term comes from the Latin word "palliare" meaning "cloaked" or "protected," and involves care which seeks to cloak or protect the terminally ill through the alleviation of their pain or disease symptoms without curing. In playing a central role in the development of palliative care, the hospice movement has been able to profoundly address two fundamental concerns of the terminally ill: (1) the fear of pain and (2) the suffering that results from unrelieved pain and symptoms.

Michael J. McCabe, PhD, is a former Fellow-in-Ethics, Department of Neurology, Memorial Sloan-Kettering Cancer Center, New York. He is currently based in Wellington, New Zealand.

Address correspondence to: Michael J. McCabe, PhD, P.O. Box 28-004, Kelburn, Wellington, New Zealand.

Assistance from Kathleen M. Foley, MD, and Nessa Coyle, RN, Pain Service, Memorial Sloan-Kettering Cancer Center, New York, NY, was appreciated.

[Haworth co-indexing entry note]: "Ethical Issues in Pain Management." McCabe Michael J. Co-published simultaneously in *The Hospice Journal* (The Haworth Press, Inc.) Vol. 12, No. 2, 1997, pp. 25-32; and: *Ethics in Hospice Care: Challenges to Hospice Values in a Changing Health Care Environment* (ed: Bruce Jennings) The Haworth Press, Inc., 1997, pp. 25-32. Single or multiple copies of this article are available for a fee from The Haworth Document Delivery Service [1-800-342-9678, 9:00 a.m. - 5:00 p.m. (EST). E-mail address: getinfo@haworth.com].

In the strict use of the term within hospice care, palliative care begins when the following criteria have been established:

- a terminal illness has been diagnosed
- death is likely or imminent
- a curative approach to care has been abandoned (although curative medicine may also benefit from, or require, concomitant palliative care). (Jeffrey 1993, 2)

While pain and suffering are conceptually distinct, for the terminally ill they are combined because the former is often the underlying cause of the latter. Pain, defined as the result of a "highly distressful, undesirable sensation or experience ordinarily associated with a physical cause," has a mesmerizing effect in terminal illness (Callahan 1993, 91). It simply blots everything out at a critical point in a patient's narrative so that he or she cannot think or respond beyond the present moment, as Emily Dickinson poignantly describes in her poem, "Final Harvest":

> Pain—has an Element of Blank—
> It cannot recollect
> When it begun—or if there were
> A Time—when it was not—
> It has no Future—but itself—
> Its Infinite contain
> Its Past—enlightened to perceive
> New Periods—of Pain. (Stoddard 1983, 140-141)

In addition, the terminally ill may internalize many of the widespread cultural fears that are associated with diseases such as cancer or AIDS, and specifically, the fear that death from these diseases is riddled with agonizing physical pain (Munley 1983, Sontag 1989). While severe pain remains one of the most inadequately treated symptoms of advanced cancer, it is estimated that 30% of cancer patients have no pain (Galazka and Hunter in Stoddard 1983, Conolly 1989). Another very real fear associated with palliation is that patients fear they will be so "doped up" that they will lose control over their dying. Consequently a fundamental need in terminal care, and one addressed by the hospice movement, is the reassurance that, for most patients, the balance between adequate pain control and being alert is possible.

Pain, the primary symptom of terminal illness, is controllable. As Cicely Saunders points out:

> it must not be forgotten that "intractable" does not mean "impossible to relieve"; its meaning is "not easily treated." Successful treat-

ment may call for much imagination and persistence but pain can be abolished while the patient still remains alert, able to enjoy the company of those around him and often able to be up and about until his death. (Munley 1983, 20)

Thus, effective pain control is the immediate need for the dying. When it is contained, other symptoms of terminal illness can be addressed. To fail to address the pain of the dying is to misunderstand the highly subjective nature of pain and to diminish any choices the terminally ill may wish to make in preparing for their deaths. The control of pain centers around three steps: (1) a detailed assessment of the patient's condition; (2) a plan of pain management; and (3) constant evaluation and monitoring. The determination of the cause of pain involves a specific and careful history of the patient. The importance of the case history lies in the fact that, generally speaking, pain is what the patient says it is; not what the doctor believes it ought to be. The patient's perception of pain and emotional response to it are critical factors in its effective relief (Galazka and Hunter in Stoddard 1983). That is why attention is given not only to tissue damage, but also to the suffering component of the pain because both are integral parts of a patient's experience of pain. Equally, because the pain threshold and the effect of symptoms vary from patient to patient, effective palliation requires constant monitoring and adjustment of the particular drug regimen.

A fundamental principle in palliative care is that continuous pain requires continuous relief. It is very counterproductive to prescribe pain relief, as was done formerly–and sadly still is in many places–solely on an "as needed" (PRN) basis. It is more effective and easier to prevent than relieve intense pain. In terminal care, analgesic medication must be given on a regular "around the clock" (ATC) basis together with an "as needed" or "pain rescue" basis. This principle is intrinsically linked with another key factor in the alleviation of pain, namely the fear of additional pain, which can, in fact, exacerbate and increase a patient's pain. As Stoddard writes:

The fear of pain increases pain itself by geometric proportions. When severe pain is experienced and is expected to continue indefinitely, even to get worse, the patient enters into a world of horror and hopelessness that for many treated by conventional methods only ends in death. (Stoddard 1983)

The all-consuming fear of unrelieved pain is simply unnecessary. Given the state of the art of palliative care, pain can be controlled, although, in a few cases, it will be at the price of reduced consciousness. The knowledge that pain relief is eminently possible is a significant part of the comfort offered to hospice patients and their families. Better understanding of pain and methods of palliation pose a challenge to the hospice movement, both to remain aware of these developments and to use this knowledge in the education of the medical and nursing profession's care of the dying.

Undertreated pain in the dying poses a threat to the autonomy of the dying patient. Patrick Hill draws a parallel between freedom from pain and the ability to die a good death. "Untreated or inadequately treated, pain can seriously compromise, if not destroy, autonomy. When that happens, the physician can no longer treat the patient as a person anymore than he or she can hope to treat the 'total pain' of his patient." Untreated pain will necessarily impact on the integrity of the doctor-patient relationship and impact on the patient's dying (Hill 1994).

Palliative care, by definition, seeks to surround or cloak the terminally ill patient. This requires the judicious use of palliation so that the extremes of overtreatment or undertreatment of pain, and the consequent diminishment of patient autonomy, are avoided. Here the maxim that medicine is both an art and a science is demonstrated clearly.

Once a patient's pain symptoms are under control there can be renewed awareness of his or her dignity and worth as a person as well as the "freedom" to address other causes of their distress and suffering. Because physical, emotional, and spiritual symptoms are closely interwoven, the emphasis is on holistic care. It would be facile indeed to suggest that all pain is related to a troubled spirit, but equally, one is unwise to ignore the concerns of the inner world and the power of memory as very real factors in addressing the pain and distress of the terminally ill. For this reason, Cicely Saunders developed the term "total pain" to describe this holistic and comprehensive approach to suffering. This term recognizes the broad reality of pain whether it be "a consequence of loneliness, spiritual distress, inappropriate diet, or tumor growth" (Siebold 1992, 96). Just as effective management of pain cannot be achieved without reference to a patient's inner world, neither can it be achieved without reference to a patient's family. The family is best served when hospice workers remain objective and respect the fact that they are only witnessing a "brief snapshot" in this particular patient-family narrative.

This discussion would remain incomplete without addressing a final ethical concern in the application of palliative care, namely the risk of hastening death for the terminally ill.

The moral and ethical question of whether or not palliative care hastens death is, in the light of recent medical literature, an open question. Several writers argue that effective palliation does not hasten death and neither does it cause respiratory depression and may, in fact, have the ability to prolong life. According to David Cundiff:

> Some people mistakenly believe that the toxic side effects of the opioids shorten the lives of cancer patients. No one questions that opioids have side effects. However, with skilful management of opioid analgesics, including anticipation of possible adverse side effects, no evidence exists that these drugs shorten life. (Cundiff 1992, 118)

Because of the patient's ability to develop tolerance for repeated doses of opioid drugs, respiratory depression is limited in effective palliative care. While there is a deterioration in respiratory function as a person nears death, this occurs as a result of the presence of an underlying pathology, and should not be confused with respiratory distress. As Kathleen Foley argues:

> In fact, respiratory depression is not a significant limiting factor in the management of patients with pain because with repeated doses, tolerance develops to this effect, allowing for adequate treatment of patients with escalating doses without respiratory compromise. (Foley 1991, 291-92)[1]

The fundamental intent of palliation for the terminally ill is the relief of suffering through effective pain relief and symptom control. Ethicists and theologians have traditionally argued that the inherent risk in palliative care—the suppression of the respiratory system—can be justified from the perspective of the intention of the caregiver.

"Intention" distinguishes what one does in an action from what one allows to happen as the result of that action. The intention in administering narcotics for the terminally ill is to relieve pain. The *Declaration on Euthanasia* states: "In this case, of course, death is in no way intended or sought, even if the risk of it is reasonably taken; the intention is simply to relieve pain effectively, using for this purpose painkillers available to medicine" (Declaration on Euthanasia 1980). This distinction between the direct and indirect intention is known within the Catholic moral tradition and in medical ethics generally as the "principle of double effect."[2]

Richard McCormick summarizes the fourfold conditions of the principle that must be present if the necessary good is to be achieved:

1. *The Nature of the Act.* The action from which harm results is good or indifferent in itself; it is not morally wrong.

2. *The Agent's Intention.* The intention must be upright, that is, the harmful effect is sincerely not intended.
3. *The Distinction Between Means and Effects.* The harmful effect must be equally immediate causally with the good effect, for otherwise it would be a means to the good effect and would be intended.
4. *Proportionality Between the Good Effect and Bad Effect.* There must be a proportionately serious reason for allowing the side-effect to occur (McCormick 1981, 413).

When these conditions are present, any resultant "harm" that occurs is referred to as an "unintended by-product" of the action. The harm is only indirectly voluntary, and it is justified by the presence of a proportionately serious reason, specifically, the imperative to relieve unbearable pain for the terminally ill. (Medical practice provides many examples of an action that has more than one effect, such as the surgical excision of a tumor that may both save life and disable the patient.)

In palliative care, the intent is to relieve pain and not to directly cause the death of the patient. Consequently, palliative care is ethically acceptable because any unintended effects are physical and not moral. The act of palliation has two effects, alleviating pain and, in the light of recent medical literature, "possible" respiratory depression. The latter effect is not intended because the terminally patient's pain is "alleviated" by the palliation and not by his or her death. Given that, by definition, the terminally ill have a fatal pathology, the level of palliation may be titrated to effect. More positively, this principle is not a "legalistic formula" but provides an aid for discerning the ethical and moral validity of an action (Ashley and O'Rourke 1989, 187).

Thus the hallmark of hospice care, palliative care, is a practical application of the moral virtues of medicine because it seeks to alleviate pain and promote healing, in the broadest sense of both terms, through the judicious use of narcotics. Ethical palliative care helps to provide a dignified death for the terminally ill hospice patient in a way that allows for greater resolution of the complexities within the human narrative–complexities which are especially highlighted in the care of the dying.

NOTES

1. Similarly, David Outerbridge and Alan Hersh state that, "Medical studies have shown . . . that the increasing tolerance to the medication is normally accompanied by a similar tolerance to adverse side effects" (1991, 119). See also Zimmerman, J. 1986; T. Ryndes 1985, 51; M. Conolly 1989, 501; C. Saunders 1991-2,

20-21; W. Wilson et al. 1992, 949-953; L. H. Heyse-Moore, 1989. M. Ashby and B. Stoffell 1991, 1323; and S. A. Schug et al. 1992, 48.

    2. The literature on this principle is considerable. See, for example, T. J. Boyle 1991, 467-585; J. F Keenan 1993, 294-315; T. Beauchamp and J. Childress 1989, 127-134; R. Gula 1989, 270-279; B. Ashley and K. O'Rourke 1989, 184-190; and J. Mangan 1949, 41-61.

REFERENCES

Ashby, M. and Stoffell, B. Therapeutic Ratio and Defined Phases: Proposal of Ethical Framework for Palliative Care *British Medical Journal* 302, 1 June 1991:1322-1324.

Ashley, B. & O'Rourke, K. *Healthcare Ethics: A Theological Analysis* St. Louis: The Catholic Health Association, 1989. Third edition.

Beauchamp, T. and Childress, J. *Principles of Biomedical Ethics* New York: Oxford University Press, 1989. Third edition.

Boyle, T.J. (Ed.). "Double Effect: Theoretical Function and Bioethical Implications," *The Journal of Medicine and Philosophy* 16 October 1991, 467-585.

Callahan, D. *The Troubled Dream of Life: Living with Mortality,* New York: Simon and Schuster, 1993.

Conolly, M. "Alternative to Euthanasia: Pain Management" *Issues in Law & Medicine* 4 (1989) 497-507.

Cundiff, D. *Euthanasia is Not the Answer: A Hospice Physician's View* New Jersey: Humana Press, 1992.

Declaration on Euthanasia Vatican City: Vatican Polyglot Press, 1980.

Foley, K. The Relationship of Pain and Symptom Management to Patient Requests for Physician-Assisted Suicide, *Journal of Pain and Symptom Management* 6, July 1991:289-297.

Gula, R. *Reason Informed by Faith* New York: Paulist Press, 1989.

Heyse-Moore, L.H. "Symptom Control in Palliative Medicine: An Update" *The British Journal of Medical Practice* 43 (August 1989). Reprint.

Hill, T.P. "Freedom From Pain: A Matter of Rights?" *Cancer Investigation,* 12,4, 1994.

Jeffrey, D. *"There Is Nothing More I Can Do!" An Introduction to the Ethics of Palliative Care* Cornwall: The Patten Press, 1993.

Keenan, J.F. "The Function of The Principle of Double Effect," *Theological Studies* 54 (1993) 294-315.

Outerbridge, D. and Hersh, A. *Easing The Passage* New York: Harper Perennial, 1991.

Mangan, J. "An Historical Analysis of the Principle of Double Effect" *Theological Studies* 10 (1949) 41-61.

McCormick, R. *How Brave a New World? Dilemmas in Bioethics* Washington: Georgetown University Press, 1981.

Munley, A. *The Hospice Alternative. A New Context for Death and Dying* New York: Basic Books, 1983.

Ryndes, T. "Psychosocial Principles of Pain Management in the Terminally Ill," in Karen Gardner, ed., *Quality of Care for the Terminally Ill: An Examination of the Issues* Chicago: Joint Commission on Accreditation of Hospitals, 1985, 46-53.

Saunders, C. "The Evolution of Hospices" *Free Enquiry* Winter 1991-92:19-23.

Schug, S.A. et al., Pharmacological Management of Cancer Pain *Drugs* 43 (1992) 44-53.

Siebold, C. *The Hospice Movement: Easing Death's Pains* New York: Twayne Publishers, 1992.

Sontag, S. *Illness As Metaphor* London: Penguin Books, 1979.

_____. *AIDS And Its Metaphors* London: Penguin Press, 1989.

Stoddard, S. *The Hospice Movement: A Better Way of Caring for the Dying* New York: Basic Books, 1983.

Wilson, W. et al., "Ordering and Administration of Sedatives and Analgesics During the Withholding and Withdrawal of Life Support From Critically Ill Patients," *JAMA* 267, 19 February 1992:949-953.

Zimmerman, J. *Hospice: Complete Care for the Terminally Ill* Baltimore: Urban and Schwarzenberg, 1986. Second edition.

Focus on the Nurse:
Ethical Dilemmas
with Highly Symptomatic Patients
Dying at Home

SUMMARY. Some serious issues face the inexperienced nurse who has the responsibility for either providing the care or directing the care of symptomatic patients dying at home. Inexperience in such care, and lack of competent medical support, can result in the nurse perceiving "ethical dilemmas" in practices which are, in reality, part of good and ethical palliative care. *[Article copies available from The Haworth Document Delivery Service: 1-800-342-9678. E-mail address: getinfo@haworth.com]*

Although most end-of-life care can be provided at home in an effective and reasonable "low tech" manner, there are a group of highly symptomatic patients who require a considerable level of both skill and technology to control symptoms at end-of-life. Nurses responsible for overseeing such care in the home are confronted with particular stresses, especially if they

---

Nessa Coyle, RN, MS, is Director of the Supportive Care Program, Pain Service, Department of Neurology at Memorial Sloan-Kettering Cancer Center.

Address correspondence to: Nessa Coyle, RN, MS, Department of Neurology, Pain Service, Memorial Sloan-Kettering Cancer Center, 1275 York Avenue, New York, NY 10021.

[Haworth co-indexing entry note]: "Focus on the Nurse: Ethical Dilemmas with Highly Symptomatic Patients Dying at Home." Coyle, Nessa. Co-published simultaneously in *The Hospice Journal* (The Haworth Press, Inc.) Vol. 12, No. 2, 1997, pp. 33-41; and: *Ethics in Hospice Care: Challenges to Hospice Values in a Changing Health Care Environment* (ed: Bruce Jennings) The Haworth Press, Inc., 1997, pp. 33-41. Single or multiple copies of this article are available for a fee from The Haworth Document Delivery Service [1-800-342-9678, 9:00 a.m. - 5:00 p.m. (EST). E-mail address: getinfo@haworth.com].

33

are inexperienced in one or another area of patient need. For example, the nurse may have the necessary technical skills but lack experience and expertise in how to apply those skills to the situation at hand. In other instances, the nurse may be very skilled in compassionate care of the dying, but feel overwhelmed and inadequate in the face of technological equipment. A nurse's inexperience in dealing with the situation at hand can result in perceived "ethical dilemmas" which may be a reflection of inexperience and nurse distress, rather than the actual situation itself. In the changing health care climate, with earlier hospital discharges, limited resources, and sicker patients being cared for at home, nurses with limited experience in palliative care may, in increasing numbers, be expected to oversee the care of these very sick patients in the home. The situation is compounded when expert resources are lacking for the nurse or the more experienced nurse feels "hampered" by those medically responsible for the patient. The prescribing home care physician, for example, if a generalist, may have limited experience in the management of refractory symptoms in the dying and be uncomfortable at prescribing the necessary doses to achieve symptom control. The nurse, who in this situation may have the most knowledge, may also have the least power.

The necessity to monitor and evaluate symptom severity and distress on a 24 hour basis, to pay attention to signs of family fatigue or irritability, and the self monitoring of one's own competence, fatigue and level of stress are an ongoing challenge for any nurse. However, the additional responsibility for guiding the care of a home death needs specific skills and calls forth ethical considerations. Evaluating the course of a home death, what went right and what went wrong, implicitly includes whether the ethical principles of respect for the person (autonomy), beneficence, non-maleficence and justice were met. "Respect for Person" recognizes the individual as an autonomous agent and protects the individual with diminished autonomy. The concepts of beneficence and non-maleficence imply, respectively, that one ought to promote good, and one ought not to inflict evil or harm. Justice deals with the concept of fairness and reflects policy and distribution of goods and services.

Ethical conflicts for nurses who are responsible for end-of-life care usually do not challenge these accepted ethical principles. The nature of their work is directed toward realizing the values of these principles. However, seeking the good of beneficence, that is, the merciful relief of pain and symptoms, may hasten death, and thereby inflict (in the mind of the inexperienced palliative care nurse) "harm" on the patient. This possible violation of the value of non-maleficence (even if not intentional) causes concern and distress to some, and adds to the considerable onus of responsibility felt by the nurse, especially the inexperienced nurse, responsible for end-of-life care in the home.

THE PATIENTS, THE SETTING, AND THE NURSES' POSITION

Advances in technology and medical care have changed the trajectory of dying. In the past death tended to be quick, often sudden, and not a long, drawn out affair. Today, death is frequently associated with a progressive debilitating predromal terminal phase. Patients are the sickest they have ever been, their dying often associated with multiple organ failure, metabolic abnormalities and blood dyscrasias. Symptoms may be multiple and require close monitoring and a high level of expertise for their control.

A percentage of these highly symptomatic dying patients choose, nowadays, to die at home. In the past, such terminal care was provided within a hospital, where the burden of care was shared. The patient was bathed, sheets changed and laundered, food provided, and comfort given by a team of auxiliary and professional staff. Each was responsible and accountable for the patient's well-being for limited periods of time. An on-site medical team helped to sort out problems and to make medical decisions. Nurses performed only the tasks for which they were trained and competent. The family could just be the family.

With the decision to die at home, however, the scenario is much different. There are limited numbers of people to share the burden and responsibility for care. Caregiver's fatigue and exhaustion creep in, with the potential of compromising end-of-life care. The nurse becomes the front-line person, essentially alone in the day to day responsibility of symptom assessment and control and family support. Although a team is within telephone reach, the feeling of support and shared responsibility for the nurse is considerably less. When things go well there is a sense of achievement, but when things do not go well and symptoms are not well controlled, the nurse feels responsible and "wanting" and, if training and experience are lacking, this indeed may be the case.

The accurate assessment of symptoms is frequently difficult in situations where there are multiple confounding factors. The patient may be a poor descriptor and magnify each symptom so that the multiple, potentially serious yet reversible problems are difficult to sort out and their worsening may be missed. The family may be highly anxious and exhausted, and either wish for a rapid death or want death forestalled "no matter what." The nurse may need to depend on the accuracy of a family's report of symptoms and effectiveness of relief strategies if the patient is non-verbal. There is always the need for an accurate assessment by the nurse. Each assessment is followed by a judgment of what intervention would be in the best interest of the patient. An inadequate assessment can lead to inappropriate actions and the patient can be harmed, as, for example, when an impending spinal cord compression is not recognized, or when the wrong drugs are prescribed in the wrong amounts. When "high tech" care is needed in the home, assessments and decisions may seem even more difficult as there is one more area as a focus for potential problems.

REFRACTORY SYMPTOMS AND LACK OF EXPERTISE IN THEIR MANAGEMENT

Intractable or refractory symptoms such as pain, dyspnea, nausea and vomiting, and an agitated delirium may accompany death in up to 25% of the terminally ill. Some of the patients are now choosing to die at home, and this places an added responsibility and burden on the home care nurse. A personal struggle of confidence may be involved, "Am I up to the job? Can I ensure a good death? Will I make a mistake?" Sometimes the nurse finds him/herself in a situation for which he/she feels neither adequately trained nor prepared. For example, a nurse with "high tech" skills may be asked to work with a patient and family because of the refractory nature of the symptoms and the requirement for parenteral infusions of highly potent drugs for their control. The nurse may have been trained to care for patients for whom the primary goal was to cure disease and preserve life. A highly cautious approach to these drugs may have been an important part of his/her training. When caring for a highly symptomatic, dying patient requiring large doses of opioids or sedative parenteral drugs to control the symptoms, such a nurse may struggle with conflicts over the "end" of controlling symptoms, and the "means" which may hasten death. Resolution of this training/experience conflict is essential–both outcomes weigh on the conscience of the nurse. In contrast, sometimes a hospice-trained nurse is asked to care for a dying patient with "high tech" needs, and feels inadequate to monitor such care. Experience in end-of-life care does not ensure adequate skill to manage complex or refractory symptoms.

In all of this, the nurse is the ongoing witness to the success or failure of the care of the patient and the support of the family. If symptoms are not well controlled, and the "unexpected" not successfully handled, the person who frequently feels the burden of guilt and responsibility is the nurse. This "burden of guilt and responsibility" is felt doubly so when the nurse is neither experienced nor adequately supported.

The following two cases illustrate the particular challenges encountered by home care nurses striving to provide competent, caring "high tech" end-of-life care within the spirit of these ethical principles. In both cases, fear of hastening death was a concern for the nurse. Although each death was different, and each family constellation unique, there were patterns and similarities which are applicable to home care end-of-life issues nurses confront routinely. Their complexity underlines the importance of skill, experience and competent medical support.

The first case is one of inexperience and lack of expertise in a specific area. It illustrates the dilemma of a nurse who had the necessary technical skills to provide good symptom control to a dying patient at home, but lacked the experience and expertise to apply those skills with confidence to the situation at hand.

> Mrs. S. was a 53 year old married hospital administrator, and mother of three, with advanced colon cancer, bilateral hydronephrosis, and lung and liver metastasis. Her major symptoms were severe abdominal pain, nausea and a high level of anxiety. She was obstructed, had a draining gastrostomy, a central access device for nutrition, and a subcutaneous opioid infusion to control her pain. Mrs. S. wanted to go home, at least for a period before her death, but became increasingly anxious and apprehensive about trusting her family to manage the tubes, technology and medication schedule on which her pain and other symptom control as well as nutrition depended. Negotiation with her managed care case manager resulted in approval for around-the-clock professional nursing care for a one month "transitional" period. During this period it was expected that her disease and symptoms would either progress or stabilize, that her family would become more comfortable in handling the technological aspects of her care, and that she, in turn, would become reassured about their capability to do this.
>
> Once home, Mrs. S's disease progressed rapidly. She experienced periodic acute pain flares, which were rapidly brought under control, and occasional episodes of nausea. Her major lasting symptom, anxiety, was difficult to control despite the use of both anxiolytics and relaxation techniques. During the last two weeks of her life, total parenteral nutrition (TPN) had been discontinued at her request. She continued with a subcutaneous infusion of an opioid, and one week prior to death, was receiving intravenous lorazepam at 3 mg per hour for the sedation she requested. Rapid adjustments of her medications in response to symptoms enabled this woman to experience first hand the reality of what had been promised her, a system that would respond rapidly to her needs. This rapid adjustment in pharmacology

and routes of administration was possible because of the 24 hour access the home care nurse had to a palliative care nurse practitioner with both the knowledge, authority, and medical backup to make these changes. The family members were clear about the goals of care, and comfortable with the approach to symptom control. They had been part of the decision making process from the beginning. The home care nurse, however, was not experienced in caring for such a highly symptomatic patient dying at home. In addition, she was unfamiliar with the doses of lorazepam in combination with opioids that were being used to control symptoms. She had not been adequately prepared for this experience, and although she adjusted the medications as asked, she was fearful that the patient's death was being hastened. This concern only became apparent when she was asked by the palliative care nurse practitioner how she was doing. She responded tearfully, expressing her worry that she was hastening this woman's death. Careful and ongoing clarification of the patient's extent of disease, content of her Living Will, goals of care, and the principle of "double effect" made the home care nurse's ongoing care of this patient and support of the family easier. In retrospect, aspects of this patient's symptom management, and the home nurse's comfort with them, should have been addressed prior to involvement with the patient. Because this had not been done, the nurse felt herself placed in an ethical dilemma: the patient's right for symptom control, on the one hand, and the nurse's own fear of hastening death on the other.

In this situation, there was a discordance in what the nurse had learned in general about the safe use and parameters for these drugs, and what was needed for the care and control of symptoms in this particular patient. The nurse followed directions but lacked understanding. This led to her sense of uncertainty and ethical conflict. Until the concerns of the nurse were recognized and addressed, there was no way in which she could address the anxiety of the family. She had not been educated about the safe and correct use of these drugs within the setting of end-of-life care. Her sense of turmoil was caused by inadequate education concerning the correct use of these drugs, coupled with a fear of doing harm.

The second case illustrates the dilemma for the nurse, who must rely on accurate family reports of symptoms and the adequacy of symptom control when the dying patient can no longer speak for him or herself.

A 54 year old man, with recently diagnosed advanced pancreatic cancer, was admitted to the hospital for stent placement. Although diagnosed only three weeks prior to admission, he had rapidly advancing disease, and was jaundiced and urticaric associated with common bile duct obstruction. He complained of mild to moderate abdominal pain which was easily managed with controlled released morphine sulphate every 8 hours, and a combination Oxycodone/ acetaminophen product which he used for "rescue doses" on an average of two to three times per day. No further anti-tumor treatment was available to him that would cure or slow down the disease.

The patient talked very openly about his dying and identified specific short term goals: (1) To say his good-byes to family and friends; (2) to make sure that he had left no "loose ends" behind for others to clear up; (3) to be pain free; and (4) to die quickly once he had "taken care of business."

He continued to talk incessantly about dying and not wanting it to be a drawn out affair. He spoke of having completed certain projects connected to his work which were important to him, of having selected a "competent individual" to continue ongoing projects, and of having completed "unfinished business" with his family (a mother, wife, and two adult daughters). The patient was very involved in planning his own terminal care. For example, he selected a hospice program in the community to provide home care as needed, prepared a carefully worded Living Will, appointed his wife to act as his health care proxy, asked which physician would sign his death certificate, made funeral arrangements, and requested that the Supportive Care Program of the Pain Service at the center where he was receiving treatment to continue to manage his pain and other symptoms.

Immediately prior to discharge he had an acute gastro-intestinal bleed, his Hct dropped to 19.4 with a Hgb of 6.5. He complained of lightheadedness, and shortness of breath, and was transfused with 2 Units of blood. This was the extent of the treatment he desired, and according to his wishes and that of his family was discharged home the following day. His abdominal pain escalated during this period and he was no longer able to tolerate oral opioids. Utilizing an already-in-place venous access device, the patient was started on an intravenous infusion of morphine initially at 2 mg/hr with 2 mg "rescues" every 15 minutes as needed. He continued on parenteral anxiolytics.

Three days following discharge the patient became febrile, developed acute shortness of breath, had evidence of further gastro-intestinal bleeding, and complained of increasing abdominal pain. He continued to talk incessantly about dying: "I have said my good-byes, I am ready to die, now I can die, why am I not dead." His acute shortness of breath (felt to have a multifactorial etiology) was relieved by oxygen, anxiolytics and increasing doses of morphine. During the three days following discharge, the patient's morphine infusion was increased from 5 mg to 26 mg/hr with "rescue" doses of 26 mg every 15 minutes as needed via PCA. He was sleeping most of the time but became acutely distressed if awake, asking "Am I not dead?" During the last 24 hours of his life the morphine infusion was increased to 40mg/hr in response to indications of abdominal discomfort as reported by his family. "Rescue" doses of 26 mg every 15 minutes as needed were available via the PCA mode and were used frequently. The patient's wife pressed the "rescue" button whenever he stirred or moaned and continued with the parenteral anxiolytics around the clock.

The patient died at home on the fourth day after discharge. His family felt they had granted him his wish, that of spending his last days at home with those he loved. They talked of the importance of it "not being a drawn out affair," as his father had died of pancreatic cancer ten years before and that had been a difficult death. In addition, his grandfather had been chronically ill and had "pulled down" the family. A daughter remarked, "Father couldn't teach us how to grow old but could teach us how to die, and he did."

The concern of the nurse, who was adjusting medications based on the family report of escalating pain, was that the goal of the family was to hasten this phase of his dying, and that she might have been coerced unwittingly to participate in this plan.

DISCUSSION

It is not only the patient one has to be concerned about in end-of-life care provided at home, but also the family, others emotionally close to the patient, and home care staff. Although the manner of death and potential symptom constellation can be predicted for many patients, for some it cannot. Family members and staff may feel, in the abstract, that they can manage any situation, but when reality strikes, many become overwhelmed, the demands made being in excess of the family's physical and emotional strength and general capabilities, and of the home care staff's experience and capabilities. Symptoms which cause the most distress for patient, family and staff alike, unless well managed, are: intractable pain, dyspnea, delirium, nausea and vomiting and severe anxiety.

Sometimes a home death is not possible or best for the patient or family, and the patient is best cared for in an inpatient hospice setting or in a hospital that cares for the dying. If it is fixed in the mind of the family and health care team that a home death is the measure of success and a hospitalized death the measure of failure when caring for the terminally ill, dying patients may be kept at home at all costs even to the detriment of themselves and of their families. When symptoms are not well controlled, or the family has inadequate physical support, the dying period may seem unending. Sadly, a rapid death becomes the hoped-for goal, while quality-of-life until death and the ability to get pleasure from a moment or a day is lost. What could have been a life-fulfilling experience becomes instead a life-draining one.

In some situations the nurse has the necessary knowledge and expertise to adjust medications or route of administration to control the troublesome symptom, but lacks the necessary authority and power to make the appropriate changes. This places the home care nurse in the untenable position of knowing how to relieve the distress of a patient but not having the necessary power to do so.

If a death at home was not peaceful, the nurse as well as the family can be left troubled, feeling that if she had been a little more skillful, had brought a symptom under control a little more promptly, paid a little more attention to a family member's observations, or somehow had fought a little bit harder to overcome financial or insurance issues to get extra help in the house, then the outcome would have been different. There is always the knowledge that for "this patient" one cannot re-do the death, but the hope is that what we can learn from the experience of this death will help patients in the future.

Legal Requirements for Confidentiality in Hospice Care

Anne M. Dellinger

SUMMARY. In the absence of federal legislation or a federal constitutional right to medical privacy, state law governs hospice workers' legal obligations. States differ in the breadth and clarity of their law, how strongly they encourage preservation of confidentiality, what aspects of a medical encounter are confidential, and when a patient is deemed to have waived the right. All states, however, recognize a legal duty of confidentiality in certain circumstances, but also recognize exceptions to the duty. Understanding the law is necessary but not sufficient; hospice staff should be prepared to adjust procedures and physical surroundings to protect confidentiality. *[Article copies available from The Haworth Document Delivery Service: 1-800-342-9678. E-mail address: getinfo@haworth.com]*

Anyone nursing the sick is soon aware of secrets and vulnerabilities of the patient and those around her.[1] This is particularly true in hospice. Hos-

Anne M. Dellinger, JD, is Professor of Public Law and Government, The University of North Carolina at Chapel Hill; formerly, Counsel, Hogan & Hartson, Washington, DC.

Address correspondence to: Anne M. Dellinger, the Institute of Government, UNC CH, C.B.#3330, Chapel Hill, NC 27599-3330.

The generosity of the following hospice staff members in sharing their experiences is gratefully acknowledged: Marisette Broadney, Palmetto Hospice, Columbia, SC; Rose Lucas, Hospice for the Carolinas, Raleigh, NC; and Marion Taylor, Hospice of Greensboro, Greensboro, NC.

[Haworth co-indexing entry note]: "Legal Requirements for Confidentiality in Hospice Care." Dellinger, Anne M. Co-published simultaneously in *The Hospice Journal* (The Haworth Press, Inc.) Vol. 12, No. 2, 1997, pp. 43-48; and: *Ethics in Hospice Care: Challenges to Hospice Values in a Changing Health Care Environment* (ed: Bruce Jennings) The Haworth Press, Inc., 1997, pp. 43-48. Single or multiple copies of this article are available for a fee from The Haworth Document Delivery Service [1-800-342-9678, 9:00 a.m. - 5:00 p.m. (EST). E-mail address: getinfo@haworth.com].

pice workers join a circle of intimates that will soon be broken–a circumstance that encourages revelations, confessions, efforts at reconciliation and final declarations. Hospice staff witness these events and from time to time are actively involved in them. Among the staff's most serious professional tasks is that of judging when to keep silent about their knowledge.

Consider these examples–each one a situation in which a hospice worker must decide whether to honor confidentiality. A patient with AIDS, being cared for at home, asks the staff not to tell his parents what the illness is. A family's lawyer asks a nurse to check patient records to see whether the patient was clearheaded in her last weeks. A patient confides to a volunteer that he's still using crack cocaine. An exhausted elderly caregiver hints that he may end his wife's life and his own. Teachers of a child whose parent recently died in the hospice program call the team social worker to discuss counseling for the child and the best grade placement. A new patient's minister greets a hospice nurse warmly–"I know you. You're caring for Mrs. Smythe too, aren't you?"

Such incidents occur frequently, causing staff to reflect on what it means to keep faith with patients and families. Confidentiality in hospice is complex because there may be tension between moral principles, because medical judgments are sometimes involved, and because the law is somewhat unclear. This paper identifies the basic legal principles and a number of recognized exceptions to the principles.

The following, apparently contradictory, comments from three legal writers illustrate the challenge in summarizing the law of medical confidentiality.

> A patient's right to privacy and confidentiality has one of the highest priorities in our system. . . . No longer is privacy and confidentiality merely a moral, ethical, professional obligation; it is a legal duty. (Hirsch 1995, 312)

> While doctors and patients agree on the desirability of confidentiality, American law is frankly ambiguous. The majority of states have no general statutory right to confidentiality of medical records, and the group of cases upholding a cause of action against providers for improper disclosure is quite small. (Dellinger 1990, 553)

> I am prepared to argue that, in terms of the number of people and the number of institutions that have routine access to identifiable medical records, medical records may be the most widely circulated personal record of any record about you. . . . They are not confidential. (Gellman 1995, 1045)

One reason for the quite divergent views expressed above is the absence of broad federal legislation on medical privacy. (A federal statute has long been expected and several groups are now drafting bills.) The highest legal arbiter, the United States Supreme Court, has not recognized privacy or confidentiality in medical treatment as a constitutional right.[2] Still, there is some federal guidance. The Medicare program's hospice regulations do address privacy issues briefly. Most importantly, the regulations require that nursing and physician services be provided "in a manner consistent with accepted standards of practice" (42 CFR §418.50). As a result, since confidentiality is widely accepted by health professionals as standard practice, confidentiality is, by implication, required by Medicare. In addition, the regulations require that clinical records be safeguarded against unauthorized use (42 CFR §418.74) and that hospice inpatient facilities offer patients and families some degree of privacy (42 CFR §418.100).

Because medical privacy is not a federal constitutional right, and there is no significant federal legislation, the states may deal with the issue as they wish. Nearly all states protect to some degree the principle of patient confidentiality, but the law of every state expresses the principle differently. All but one state, for example, recognizes a doctor-patient testimonial privilege; that is, an assumption that a patient's doctor should not testify in court against him. However, the states differ in how extensive and clear their law is on this subject, how strongly they encourage health providers to maintain confidentiality, what aspects of a medical encounter they regard as confidential, and when they consider a patient to have waived the privilege of keeping his medical status private. Instructions for handling knowledge about a person's HIV status or AIDS also varies. Many states regulate this medical information by statute or administrative regulation.

Likewise, the reasons a state recognizes for not preserving confidentiality vary. Perhaps the most common exception is the one for reporting child abuse or neglect. Wherever a medical professional practices, she should assume such information is probably not confidential. Furthermore, if she begins to suspect abuse or neglect, she should immediately verify the assumption as to the law and then, if necessary, report the suspicion.

Some states have few statutes or regulations that direct medical professionals to protect or breach confidentiality in specific instances. In that case, law on the subject may still be found in judicial opinions, administrative regulations, Attorney-General opinions or other sources. Because the law of confidentiality is peculiar to each state and careful legal research may be required to uncover it, hospice administrators usually need assistance in mastering the law. If a hospice program has access to counsel, a lawyer could be useful in training staff and thereafter in answering especially difficult questions. If legal services are not regularly available to a program, the state and national hospice organizations may be able to advise and provide or recommend written materials.

In most jurisdictions, the following procedures would be prudent means of safeguarding confidentiality and meeting legal requirements.

A hospice program should not identify its patients to outsiders. While this is always good practice, a health care provider runs a serious legal risk if he identifies a patient when doing so also discloses significant medical information about the patient. Thus, an abortion clinic or AIDS treatment facility, a hospice program (because a terminal diagnosis is a condition of entry) or tuberculosis hospital is more likely to be liable for identifying patients than would a general hospital. On this principle, the friendly minister mentioned above should be answered with a pleasant greeting but no comment on whether the hospice nurse is serving Mrs. Smythe.

The understanding that staff members' first duty is to the patient, and that the duty includes confidentiality, answers some but not all of providers' questions. (The primary focus on the patient should be restated occasionally in hospice training, since it is so often said that the family is the unit of care in hospice.) The example of an AIDS patient who asked that his parents not be told his diagnosis shows the need for judgment and flexibility in handling confidentiality issues. If his parents were not also his caretakers, or the disease were not communicable, the patient's wish should be respected. Staff would normally honor, for example, a patient's request that a friend or relative be told little or nothing about his condition. For an AIDS patient's caregivers, however, ignorance would be dangerous. A number of courts have held that medical professionals may, and in some circumstances, must reveal patients' secrets when necessary to prevent harm to others.[3]

Therefore, the program would normally have a legal duty to inform the parents of their son's condition and train them in precautions. Similarly, most courts and legal commentators view information that the patient is at risk as creating an exception to confidentiality. In the cases of the patient using cocaine and the woman whose husband is tempted to hasten her death, the confidences should not be kept because the patients' welfare is threatened.

Exceptions to confidentiality are also recognized for auditing care, for research, law enforcement, criminal prosecution, and civil litigation purposes. For requests in the latter three categories, however, the health provider should respond only to a subpoena or a warrant and it would often be prudent for the program to seek a court order before releasing information.

In the other examples given, a hospice worker would want more information before making the requested disclosures. Whom exactly does the "family lawyer" represent? If she is the legally designated agent (a representation that the hospice should verify) of the former patient's executor or next of kin, and is requesting records on that person's behalf, she would normally have a right of access to the patient's records. Even so, a hospice worker would be wise not to comment casually on whether the patient was "clearheaded"–a label with obvious implications for the validity of wills and gifts made during life. Likewise, before discussing a former patient's child, a social worker would need consent from the child's parent or guardian.

Understanding the law is only the first step toward achieving a satisfactory level of confidentiality in a hospice program. Administrators and caregivers must also be willing to adjust procedures and physical surroundings. For example, a nurse visiting in a home should ask for privacy before responding to calls from or about other patients. If the hospice program's office is in a building shared with other tenants, is open for tours or sometimes used by the public, the paging and message systems, posted lists of patients and any other potential source of inadvertent disclosures must be managed appropriately. Some hospice programs go further than the law requires. At a patient's request, they have taken such steps as having staff members park at some distance from a home, wear ordinary clothing for visits, or omit discussion of a particular patient in case presentations made to hospice staff. Whatever efforts a program chooses to undertake, what is essential is that each staff member and volunteer be thoroughly trained in confidentiality as an important aspect of patient care and then reminded regularly that it is legally required of all medical providers.

NOTES

1. See, Burnum, John F., "Secrets About Patients," 324 *New Eng. J. of Med.* 1130 (April 18, 1991).

2. A case from the 1995-96 Term of the Supreme Court could revisit this point. The case, Jaffee v. Redmond, No. 95-266, directly concerns the existence of a psychotherapist-patient privilege under the Federal Rules of Evidence.

3. The best known decision is *Tarasoff v. Regents of the University of California,* 17 Cal. 3d 425, 551 P.2d 334 (1976).

REFERENCES

Hirsch, H.L., "Disclosure about patients," *Legal Medicine.* (3d Ed.) American College of Legal Medicine. Mosby: St. Louis, 1995, 312.

Dellinger, A.M. "Medical Records," in Dellinger, A.M. (Ed.) *Healthcare Facilities Law.* Little, Brown, & Co.: Boston, 1990, 553.

Gellman, R.M., quoted in "Health Facilities Should Take Steps to Protect Privacy, Conference Told," *BNA's Health Law Reporter* (July 6, 1995) 1045.

The Role of the Physician in Hospice

Barry M. Kinzbrunner

SUMMARY. As the concept of hospice has evolved in the United States, it has become apparent that there is a significant need for increased physician participation in all aspects of the care of terminally ill patients provided by hospice programs. Four distinct physician roles have emerged: the attending physician, the consulting physician, the hospice medical director, and the hospice team physician. As the roles of the hospice medical director and team physician have become better defined, many physicians are finding that palliative medicine and full time hospice employment is a rewarding career option. The increased involvement of physicians in all aspects of hospice and palliative care will result in measurable improvement in the quality of patient care that hospice programs provide to terminally ill patients and families. *[Article copies available from The Haworth Document Delivery Service: 1-800-342-9678. E-mail address: getinfo@haworth. com]*

In the early years of hospice in the United States, physician participation was extremely limited for a number of reasons. While all would agree that physicians serve as patient advocates, physicians have traditionally

Barry M. Kinzbrunner, MD, FACP, is Vice President/National Medical Director for Vitas Healthcare Corporation.

Address correspondence to: Barry M. Kinzbrunner, MD, Vice President/National Medical Director, Vitas Healthcare Corporation, 100 S. Biscayne Blvd. 17th Floor, Miami, FL 33131.

The author would like to gratefully acknowledge the participation and support of Vitas Healthcare Corporation and The Hastings Center.

[Haworth co-indexing entry note]: "The Role of the Physician in Hospice." Kinzbrunner, Barry M. Co-published simultaneously in *The Hospice Journal* (The Haworth Press, Inc.) Vol. 12, No. 2, 1997, pp. 49-55; and: *Ethics in Hospice Care: Challenges to Hospice Values in a Changing Health Care Environment* (ed: Bruce Jennings) The Haworth Press, Inc., 1997, pp. 49-55. Single or multiple copies of this article are available for a fee from The Haworth Document Delivery Service [1-800-342-9678, 9:00 a.m. - 5:00 p.m. (EST). E-mail address: getinfo@haworth.com].

been viewed as the final arbiter of determining what is best for the patient. This challenges one of the fundamental tenets of hospice care, that the patient should make the ultimate decisions regarding the medical care that they receive. The autonomy and independence of physicians in providing patient care was put in question by the interdisciplinary team approach to care espoused by hospices (Kurtz 1988). The standard medical school curriculum does not place great emphasis on the principles of palliative care (Corless 1983, Rhymes 1990, Bulkin and Lukashok 1988) in the treatment of the terminally ill, and tends to promulgate the attitude among physicians that patient mortality is a form of failure (Braverman 1991, Slevins et al. 1990). In spite of these barriers, physician involvement in hospice is vital, and is underscored by the Medicare Hospice Benefit (Medicare Hospice Regulations 1993), which defines the role of the patient's attending physician while mandating, as a condition of participation, that hospices provide their own medical directors to oversee plans of care and ensure that patients receive appropriate medical management. In fact, as hospices have evolved, four distinct physician roles have emerged: the attending physician, the consulting physician, the hospice medical director, and the hospice team physician (Hadlock 1983, Ajemian 1993, Kinzbrunner 1993, Academy of Hospice Physicians 1993a).

ATTENDING PHYSICIAN

Defined by the Medicare Hospice Benefit as a doctor of medicine or osteopathy who "is identified by the individual, at the time he or she elects to receive hospice care, as having the most significant role in the determination of the individual's medical care," (Medicare Hospice Regulations 1993) the attending physician is a key member of the hospice interdisciplinary team. It is this physician, in conjunction with the hospice medical director, who is required to certify that the patient has a prognosis of 6 months or less, and is, therefore, eligible for the Medicare Hospice Benefit (Medicare Hospice Regulations 1993, Brody and Lynn 1984). Knowing more about the patient's illness, prior treatments, and current state of ill health than other members of the hospice team, the attending physician's expertise, care, and guidance helps ensure that the patient receives quality palliative care.

Attending physicians vary in their degree of active participation in the ongoing care of their hospice patients. Many physicians continue to remain very involved with their patients, continuing to manage their symptoms with the aid of the hospice interdisciplinary team and periodically visiting with their patients either in the office or at home. Other physicians choose a less active role, functioning primarily in an advisory capacity so that continuity of care is maintained (Wiest 1993), while allowing the hospice physician and the interdisciplinary team to provide for the medical needs of their patients. Regardless of the level of attending physician involvement, the special nature of the doctor-patient relationship is preserved and respected.

CONSULTING PHYSICIAN

Patients will sometimes experience symptoms that require the expertise of consultant physician specialists. For example, an orthopedist will be needed to assist in the immobilization of a pathological fracture or a pulmonologist will be requested to perform a therapeutic thoracentesis to relieve a patient's dyspnea (Hadlock 1983). As hospices in the United States have accepted the responsibility of professional patient management in order to ensure that the care being provided to the patient is consistent with principles of palliative medicine, it is incumbent upon hospices to have relationships with various consultant physicians (McKeen and Billings 1991).

Some hospices will develop relationships with several consultants, one from each of the various medical specialties, in order to meet the needs of patients under hospice care. Other hospices will develop relationships with multiple physicians representing each specialty in the community, and engage them as consultants based on individual patient need. The latter arrangement, while somewhat more cumbersome administratively, takes into account prior doctor-patient relationships between hospice patients and community consultants, and also recognizes that attending physicians often have a preference for specific specialists.

HOSPICE MEDICAL DIRECTOR AND TEAM PHYSICIAN

While the participation of attending and consulting physicians in the care of hospice patients is fairly straightforward, the role of the physicians who are directly employed by hospice programs continues to evolve. The Medicare Hospice Benefit defines the hospice medical director as a hospice employed physician "who assumes overall responsibility for the medical component of the hospice's patient care program" (Medicare Hospice Regulations 1993). While this definition seems fairly clear, as one explores how hospice medical directors fulfill their responsibilities, it is equally clear that there is significant variance from hospice to hospice.

As already discussed, physician involvement in the early years of hospice was fairly limited. Hospices would, therefore, engage a single physician, or two if they were fortunate, on a part-time basis, sometimes paid and sometimes volunteer, to provide medical direction to the interdisciplinary team. Activities might include weekly or bi-weekly meetings with the team members to develop and review patients' plans of care, ensuring that patients had prescriptions written for their medications, and, on rare occasions, making home visits. Occasionally, if time permitted, the physician might assist the hospice as a liaison and problem solver with attending physicians, and might be involved in some quality assurance activities (Hadlock 1983, Kinzbrunner 1993).

As hospice programs have grown, the need for more medical direction and support has increased markedly. For some hospices, this has meant increasing their cadre of part-time physicians, or hiring full-time medical directors to provide more support to the team, more patient home visits, and more administrative and educational activities (Academy of Hospice Physicians 1993a). For other hospices, the need for administrative, quality assurance, and educational activities was so great that it was necessary to separate them from direct patient care responsibilities, resulting in the differentiation of physician roles within those organizations (Kinzbrunner 1993).

Hospice Team Physician

The hospice team physician is the physician member of the interdisciplinary team. His or her primary focus is to ensure that all patients cared for by their team receive appropriate palliative medical care. Hospice team physicians are responsible for certifying that all patients cared for by the hospice under the Medicare Hospice Benefit have a prognosis of 6 months or less and to recertify that prognosis at appropriate intervals (Medicare Hospice Regulations 1993, Brody and Lynn 1984). In addition, they actively participate in interdisciplinary team meetings, provide patient visits at home and in hospice inpatient beds, maintain contact with attending physicians about their patients, and provide support and education to other members of the hospice patient care team (Hadlock 1983, Ajemian 1993, Kinzbrunner 1993, Academy of Hospice Physicians 1993a, Wiest 1993, Storey 1993, Vitas Healthcare Corp. 1993a).

By being devoted to direct patient care activities, the team physician is better able to positively influence pain and symptom management decisions made by attending physicians and other members of the team. The opportunity for direct physician/patient contact provided by hospice team physician visits at home or in hospice inpatient beds not only allows for more optimal pain and symptom management, but often has significant psychosocial benefits for patients and families. The value of these visits should never be underestimated! Finally, there is additional time available for the hospice physician to educate members of the hospice patient care team in pain and symptom management techniques, and they often can provide valuable staff support during times of stress (Beszterczey 1977).

Medical Director

Being relieved of responsibilities directly related to the function of the team allows the hospice medical director to focus on the medical care delivered in the hospice program as a whole. In this way, the medical director can devote attention to such activities as the evaluation of the overall quality of patient care provided by the hospice, the supervision of the hospice team physicians, education and training of hospice staff, and direct participation in administrative functions of the hospice program. They also have time available to provide increased community professional education and liaison activities, and can involve themselves in developing and participating in medical education programs and palliative care research projects (Hadlock 1983, Kinzbrunner 1993, Academy of Hospice Physicians 1993a, Vitas Healthcare Corp. 1993b, Williams 1993).

Although some of these functions may appear peripheral to daily patient management, their direct impact on patient care is very apparent. By devoting more time to quality improvement activities, medical directors are able to address specific medical challenges that are discovered within the hospice program. Medical director supervision of hospice team physicians, especially important in large hospices where many physicians are employed, ensures a consistency and provides a standard for quality pain and symptom management throughout the organization. The participation of the medical director in administrative and management activities of a hospice program provides important contributions to the maintenance of the proper balance between quality care and cost effectiveness. Medical director involvement in the training of hospice staff provides a more creative and innovative educational forum, resulting in improved staff performance at the bedside. Medical directors who participate in professional education and liaison activities increase community physicians' awareness of the principles of hospice and palliative medicine, resulting in an increase in patient/family access to hospice services. Finally, with growing interest in hospice and palliative medicine, it is the hospice medical director (and the hospice team physician) who possess the experience, knowledge, expertise, and time to develop and participate in the medical education training programs (MacLeod 1993, Academy of Hospice Physicians 1993b) and palliative care research programs (Kinzbrunner et al. 1990, Kinzbrunner and Pratt in press) that are so desperately needed in order to increase our knowledge about the care of the terminally ill. This will result in improved pain and symptom management techniques and further enhancement of the quality of life of terminally ill patients and their families.

CONCLUSION

Clearly, as hospice has evolved in the United States, there has been and continues to be a significant increase in the participation of physicians in all aspects of the care of terminally ill patients served by hospice programs. Although most hospices still employ medical directors and team physicians on a part-time basis, a recent survey performed by the Academy of Hospice Physicians revealed that 61 of 371 (13%) hospice medical directors considered themselves to be full-time employees of a hospice program (Academy of Hospice Physicians 1993b). As more physicians devote their professional careers to hospice and palliative care, and as physician role differentiation within hospices allows physicians to participate in more diverse activities, there will be measurable improvement in the quality of patient care that hospice programs deliver to their patients and families (Kinzbrunner 1993).

REFERENCES

Academy of Hospice Physicians, 1993 AHP Membership Survey Statistics, 1993a.

Academy of Hospice Physicians, Hospice Medical Practice Committee, 1993b. Role definitions for hospice medical director, associate medical director, and hospice physician.

Ajemian I: The interdisciplinary team. p. 17. In Doyle D, Hanks GWC, MacDonald N (ed): *Oxford Textbook of Palliative Medicine.* Oxford University Press, Oxford, 1993.

Beszterczey A: Staff stress on a newly-developed palliative care service, the psychiatrist's role. *Can Psychiatr Assoc J* 22:347, 1977.

Braverman AS: Medical oncology in the 1990s. *Lancet* 337:901, 1991.

Bulkin W, Lukashok H: Rx for dying: the case for hospice. *N Engl J Med* 318:376, 1988.

Brody H, Lynn J: The physician's responsibility under the new medicare reimbursement for hospice care. *N Engl J Med* 310:920, 1984.

Corless IB: The hospice movement in North America. p. 335. In Corr CA, Coor DM (ed): *Hospice Care, Principles and Practice.* Springer, New York, 1983.

Hadlock DC: Physicians roles in hospice care. p. 103. In Corr CA, Coor DM (ed): *Hospice Care, Principles and Practice.* Springer, New York, 1983.

Kinzbrunner BM, Policzer J, Miller B, Neiber N: Non-invasive pain control in the terminally ill patient. *Am J Hospice & Pall Care* 7(4):26, 1990.

Kinzbrunner BM: Hospice medical director role redefined. p. 111. In: *Innovations '93, Models for cost management and health care quality.* ACPE, Tampa, 1993.

Kinzbrunner BM, Pratt MM: Severity index scores correlate with survival of AIDS patients. *Am J Hospice & Pall Care,* in press.

MacLeod, RN: Teaching hospice medicine to medical students, house staff, and other caregivers in the United Kingdom. *The Hospice Journal* 9(1):55, 1993.

Kurtz ME: The dual role dilemma. p. 66. In Curry W (ed): *New Leadership in Health Care Management: The Physician Executive.* Lithocolor, Tampa, 1988.

McKeen E, Billings JA: Reimbursement for physician services under the medicare benefit. *Hospice Update,* December 5,1991.

Medicare Hospice Regulations, *42 Code of Federal Regulations,* Part 418, 1993.

Rhymes J: Hospice care in America. *J Am Med Assoc* 264:369, 1990.

Slevins ML, Stubbe L, Plant HJ et al.: Attitudes to chemotherapy: comparing views of patients with cancer with those of doctors, nurses, and the general public. *Brit Med J* 300:1458, 1990.

Storey P: What is the role of the hospice physician? *Am J Hospice & Pall Care* 10(6):2, 1993.

Vitas Healthcare Corp. Team physician job description, policy 9:13. *Vitas Policy Manual,* 1993a.

Vitas Healthcare Corp. Medical Director job description, policy 9:04. *Vitas Policy Manual,* 1993b.

Wiest JV: The hospice advantage. *Am J Hospice & Pall Care* 10(6):12, 1993.

Williams R: Wanted: hospice medical director, apply within. *Am J Hospice & Pall Care* 10(6):9, 1993.

The Role of Ethics Committees in Hospice Programs

Richard B. Fife

SUMMARY. Ethics committees are still relatively new to hospices, aside from those that are directly related to hospitals. This article takes a brief look at how one company formed and trained its ethics committees for several hospices providing care in the home setting. It delineates the composition of the committee, how the committee is trained, the functions of an operating committee, the various types of committees, and takes a look at the pitfalls and problems of such committees. *[Article copies available for a fee from The Haworth Document Delivery Service: 1-800-342-9678. E-mail address: getinfo@haworth.com]*

As home health and hospice organizations find themselves grappling more and more with ethical dilemmas, there is a greater need to create a structure for resolving these dilemmas. This article takes a brief look at the way that the nation's largest hospice corporation has chosen to deal with this situation. It looks at the formation of an ethics committee, its membership, functions, training and value. It mentions the problems and pitfalls of such a committee and lists the current types of hospice ethics committees. Since the hospice itself is so centered on patient care, it is appropriate to begin with a brief case study.

Richard B. Fife, DMin, is a United Methodist minister, employed by Vitas Healthcare Corporation in Miami as the Vice-President of Bioethics and Pastoral Care. He created the Department of Bioethics for the country's largest hospice system and currently is an ethicist for 30 local hospice programs.

Address correspondence to: Richard B. Fife, Vitas Healthcare Corporation, 3700 Executive Way, Miramar, FL 33025.

[Haworth co-indexing entry note]: "The Role of Ethics Committees in Hospice Programs." Fife, Richard B. Co-published simultaneously in *The Hospice Journal* (The Haworth Press, Inc.) Vol. 12, No. 2, 1997, pp. 57-63; and: *Ethics in Hospice Care: Challenges to Hospice Values in a Changing Health Care Environment* (ed: Bruce Jennings) The Haworth Press, Inc., 1997, pp. 57-63. Single or multiple copies of this article are available for a fee from The Haworth Document Delivery Service [1-800-342-9678, 9:00 a.m. - 5:00 p.m. (EST). E-mail address: getinfo@haworth.com].

CASE STUDY

When he came onto the hospice program, the patient was a 41 year old male with end stage AIDS. His pain was being managed fairly effectively with Tylenol with Codeine. His primary caregiver was his mother, who was providing the care in her home. Several times the patient had requested that he be allowed to die on his birthday surrounded by his friends. Three days prior to his 42nd birthday, the primary physician ordered that an IV morphine drip be started on the patient with an IV rate of 50mg/hr. Both the patient and his mother were aware that such a high dosage would most likely kill the patient within a short period of time. Both were supportive of the physician's order. However, the hospice RN was uncomfortable with this decision, and she brought the situation to the attention of the Team Director. The Team Director approached the Medical Director of the hospice, who confronted the primary physician. The primary physician was angry because his order was being questioned, and he stated that the patient and PCG had agreed previously to this plan and that he thought hospice was about death with dignity.

Had there not been an ethics committee in the hospice, this case would probably have ended at this point. The Medical Director would most likely accept the decision of the physician—pro or con—feeling that at least an effort was made to interject hospice philosophy. However, because there was a trained, operating ethics committee, the hospice nurse and Medical Director brought this situation before one of the gatekeepers of the committee, requesting that a meeting be immediately called into session. Input and participation was sought from the patient, the primary caregiver, hospice nurse, and primary physician. This was the rare event of a case being brought before the ethics committee without the consent of the patient and the patient's family.

THE HOSPICE ETHICS COMMITTEE

Organization

In 1991, Vitas Healthcare Corporation, the nation's largest provider of hospice care, created a Department of Bioethics in its corporate office in Miami. Among its various responsibilities a primary goal for this department was to organize and train ethics committees in all of the various regions where Vitas had operating hospices. The first committee was organized in South Florida, where three hospices existed within thirty minutes of each other. A regional committee was set up to represent the entire region. Two persons were selected by the Vice-President of Bioethics to convene the group. These persons were chosen because of their known interest in ethics.

Membership

Interdisciplinary Team. The first members were chosen from the interdisciplinary team to represent the various disciplines that work within hospice. The conveners chose nurses, chaplains, social workers, physicians, home health aides, and volunteers. People were generally chosen who were known to ask ethical questions during team meetings or around the hospice.

Management. One or two persons were selected from the managing staff. Usually the General Manager or Director of Operations was not asked to be on the committee because of concern that this might dampen the deliberations.

Community. In addition to staff members selected from the team and management, several persons were asked to serve from a community perspective. These were non-Vitas people; and, generally, they make up about one fourth of the membership of the ethics committee. These persons have included an administrator of a nursing home, an ethics professor, a minister in the community, and other persons with a concern about hospice and/or ethics. Community members are vital to a committee of this nature. Not only do they bring a differing perspective from the community served by the hospice, they also help to keep the committee honest and focused rather than becoming a discussion group.

Membership represents the various ethnic groups and sexes that make up both the staff and the patients of Vitas. The group is composed of approximately twenty persons. Such a variety and number of persons contribute to the richness of perspective in the deliberations of the committee.

Functions of the Committee

Education. During the orientation and training period, the committee is educated in ethical theory, ethical principles, the use and importance of a methodology in doing case review, and the pros and cons of various ethical issues in healthcare, such as withholding and withdrawing treatment, euthanasia and assisted suicide, informed consent and refusing treatment, advance directives and patient autonomy. Articles on these subjects are provided to committee members as a matter of course, and in-services and workshops are provided on current issues. In addition, the regional committees have set up a one day retreat every year for evaluation, continuing education and ethical reflection.

Education of Hospice Staff and Other Healthcare Providers. Committees provide regular in-services to hospice staff on ethical issues in healthcare. They also provide education through the deliberations that they make on policy issues such as CPR/DNR, withdrawal of treatment, and other concerns. In addition, some committees set up similar in-services or conferences for the nursing and group homes that have hospice patients.

Education of the Community. Committees sponsor ethics conferences for the community. In one committee an attorney on the ethics committee held a free evening seminar on living wills for the community in a local church.

Case Review. The primary concern of the ethics committee is to be patient-centered. The ethics committee is set up to function as an advisory group for ethical dilemmas relating to patients and their families. A case consultation can be held at a regular monthly meeting or a meeting can be called within 48 hours if such a need exists.

Policy Review. Committees may write guidelines or draft policies on issues such as CPR/DNR, withdrawing treatments, hospice and ventilator-appropriate patients, and other policies with ethical concerns.

Research. Some committees have the additional element of research as part of their job responsibilities. These groups may research issues or areas of concern for presentation to the hospice.

Training

Initially, Vitas contracted with a bioethics group in California to do the necessary training for all of their ethics committees in hospices in the various regions. The committees were organized to meet on a monthly basis for a period of two hours, except for the first two meetings which were designated for orientation and were three hours in duration. These first two sessions dealt with ethical theory, principles and methodology. Complete training was over a period of one year, and subsequent sessions dealt with the core curriculum and issues of hospice and ethics and practice with case studies. Workbooks were provided to all members, as were copies of relevant articles and periodicals.

Value

Perhaps the greatest value of the ethics committee has been the creation of a moral community that has been made available to discuss biomedical ethical issues on behalf of patients, families, and staff. The discussion has often helped to clarify issues of importance in patient care. Likewise, it has often given support to healthcare workers who are involved in the decision-making process. It has also been helpful in writing policies and/or clarifying guidelines for the hospice in relation to DNR, life-sustaining treatments, and other controversial subjects.

TYPES OF HOSPICE ETHICS COMMITTEES

Vitas has hospices in states as varied as California, Texas, Illinois, Florida, New Jersey, and Ohio. Ethics committees have been organized in each of these areas using a similar training and methodology for case consultation. All of the committees have developed their own guidelines and mission statement, but the similar structure, training and identical methodology have produced a similar product in each state. Wherever practical, the committees are regional in nature. For example, there is a regional committee for the hospices in Dallas, Ft. Worth and Grand Prairie, as the travel distance by car is less than an hour. On the other hand, the committees in San Antonio or Houston are local committees for the particular hospice.

The typical hospice in this country is non-profit and operates with a patient census of between 10 and 100. Perhaps 10% of these hospices have an operating ethics committee, unless they are hospital-based. The hospital-based hospice is required by the Joint Commission to have some system for redressing ethical concerns of patients and families. Generally, this requirement can be met through creating a hospice ethics committee, or by having access to the ethics committee of an affiliated hospital. Where ethics committees exist in the typical hospices they generally have received some type of orientation and training, although usually not from paid consultants on a systematic basis. These committees usually meet on a regular basis on a monthly or quarterly schedule, with a 24-48 hour emergency call basis for case consultations.

Another arrangement that works in some communities is for several small hospices to form a joint ethics committee and deal with the patient and family concerns of persons from all of the hospices. This creates a community spirit of cooperation and adds more points of view to the discussion. The disadvantages to such efforts are related to concerns about competition and confidentiality.

Rather than create their own ethics committees, some hospices that are hospital-based or nursing-home based are represented on the ethics committees of those particular institutions. There are some problems related to palliative care versus curative care as well as other concerns, but there is a common ground and great opportunities for cooperation and treating the whole patient in the same setting.

PROBLEMS AND PITFALLS

One problem related to forming an ethics committee is that of money and resources. If a consultant is hired for the training of the committee, then money must be provided for the salary and expenses of that particular individual. In addition, there would be some costs around workbooks and articles for the committee. The right persons need to be chosen to provide the leadership required to form and guide the committee. Then time must be allowed for anywhere from 12 to 20 staff members to meet on a regular basis. In addition, one must be able to secure community involvement, which is often a difficult process. To operate without community members is a pitfall for the committee, as it may turn into a staff discussion group.

In order to form a moral community capable of dealing with the issues presented in a hospice setting, it is necessary to provide a thorough and worthwhile training for the committee. Training generally takes a year, and continuing education is a part of the life of the committee. Is there enough money or knowledgeable leadership to provide the needed training? One pitfall is that many committees have a brief training period, either because of money, other resources or time factors. This will hinder the work of the committee.

Another pitfall for committees is focusing on case consultations as the only important work of the committee. Education is an extremely important function of the community, as is policy review. If the committee works to fully educate itself, the staff and the community, then there will actually be fewer case consultations brought to the committee.

Education and policy review are not very glamorous. Some committee members grow frustrated or feel that important work is not being done if cases are not brought before the committee on a regular basis.

In healthcare there is a great deal of staff turnover. Many new persons will have to be added to the ethics committee simply because of the loss of staff members. They will have to be oriented, trained and made to feel a part of the moral community. All of this takes time and resources.

One final problem or pitfall for the committee is to have an individual on the committee who is very argumentative and seeks to constantly dominate all of the proceedings at each meeting. Here a strong chairperson is needed, or fresh orientation, or term limits.

FUTURE

Hospice will feel continuing pressure to establish ethics committees from state regulations, the Joint Commission, or simply from the moral dilemmas associated with care for the terminally ill in a world of shrinking resources. A systematic approach for resolving moral dilemmas is needed; that need will be met by either a trained full committee such as Vitas initiated by policy in all of their hospices, the interdisciplinary team meeting as an ethics committee, an ethics consultant, or a hired staff person who is used full time or part time for this purpose.

Growth in Caring
and Professional Ethics in Hospice

Bernice Catherine Harper

SUMMARY. There is a continual growing concern and impetus being placed on comprehensive care and treatment of the individual
from birth to death. There is also strong evidence to lead one to believe that humanization of health care delivery must include attention
to the development of health workers who are academically, emotionally, and psychologically prepared to deal with the dying patient and
the family. Health professionals must learn to cope with anxieties arising from such experiences. This requires an adjustment period for the
professional, a time for adaption and a working through of one's own
feelings about death, dying and life's end. In other words, health professionals must come to grips with their own feelings about their own
mortality, life's end and the in-between life processes.
  This paper identifies six stages that the health professionals must
go through in learning to be comfortable in working with terminal
illnesses and catastrophic diseases. This involves the Harper Schematic Comfortability Growth and Development Scale as a conceptual
framework in learning to care for the terminally ill and dying. *[Article
copies available for a fee from The Haworth Document Delivery Service:
1-800-342-9678. E-mail address: getinfo@haworth.com]*

Bernice Catherine Harper, MSW, MScPH, LLD, is Medical Care Adviser,
Health Care Financing Administration, Department of Health and Human Services, Washington, DC. She is Chair of the National Hospice Organization's Task
Force on Access to Hospice Care by Minority Groups.
  Address correspondence to: Dr. Bernice Catherine Harper, Health Care Financing Administration, Department of Health and Human Services, Suite 403B,
200 Independence Avenue, S.W., Washington, D.C. 20201.

  The assistance of Swiger Associates, Greenville, SC is gratefully acknowledged.

  [Haworth co-indexing entry note]: "Growth in Caring and Professional Ethics in Hospice." Harper,
Bernice Catherine. Co-published simultaneously in *The Hospice Journal* (The Haworth Press, Inc.) Vol.
12, No. 2, 1997, pp. 65-70; and: *Ethics in Hospice Care: Challenges to Hospice Values in a Changing
Health Care Environment* (ed: Bruce Jennings) The Haworth Press, Inc., 1997, pp. 65-70. Single or
multiple copies of this article are available for a fee from The Haworth Document Delivery Service
[1-800-342-9678, 9:00 a.m. - 5:00 p.m. (EST). E-mail address: getinfo@haworth.com].

Ethics in hospice care must address the need for continuing professional education for caregivers and providers. Hospice providers must be technically competent, culturally sensitive, compassionate, understanding, and accepting health caregivers and providers. These characteristics are as important and necessary to quality hospice care as is specific disciplinary specialty training, such as medicine, nursing, social work, religion, and other allied health professions. In addition, training and on-going supervision are crucial and critical for home health aides and volunteers.

Hospice care lacking in behavioral knowledge and skills, relative to the psychological and psychosocial aspects of death and dying, is equivalent to the provision of inadequate and unethical medical care. Such treatment borders on malpractice. The current state of the art in the care of the dying requires that it be tailored to many settings and modalities of care, including homes, hospitals, nursing homes, and hospices. Different settings pose different problems and challenges.

Ethicists and ethics committees must take these issues into consideration in their deliberations. There can be no appropriate death without appropriate caring. But what is "caring," specifically in hospice, and how does it relate to ethics?

Caring has nothing to do with sentimentality. At the core of genuine caring lies the question: How does one give oneself totally, yet preserve oneself totally?

Care providers in the health field do not enter practice academically, intellectually, or emotionally prepared to deal with death and dying. They must learn to cope with their anxieties arising from their caring experiences. This requires an adjustment period for the care providers, a time for adaption and working through of one's own feelings about death, dying, life's end and the quality of living near death.[1]

Professional anxieties in catastrophic diseases and terminal illnesses are observable phenomena for which a coping mechanism can be developed. The care providers who are helped to come to grips with their own feelings are enabled to give strength and support to patients and relatives. The patient can be helped to die with dignity and self-respect. Families can be helped to come through a traumatic experience with some semblance of mental health. Central to this thesis is the Schematic Comfort-Ability Growth and Development Scale in coping with professional anxieties in death and dying. This scale consists of six stages (see Figure 1).

The care providers in Stage I are anxious about death; and death is threatening to their personhood. This is the stage of knowledge and anxiety. It is also known as the stage of intellectualization. Care givers in this stage mostly give tangible services to patients and families and provide

FIGURE 1. Coping with Professional Anxiety in Death and Dying

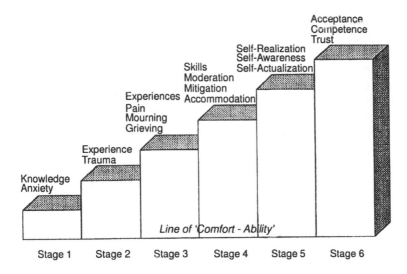

these services on an intellectual basis without in-depth feelings, as it were. Care providers also cope and manage by withdrawal; they feel concerned but are uncomfortable.

Care providers use Stage I to become familiar with the health care setting. These activities provide areas for escape from the realities of the impending, threatening situation. It is a two-pronged threat to the care providers because they must not only familiarize themselves with the health care facility, but also with the physical disease and the death and dying aspects of the patients. Thus, there is a need for an adaption and adjustment in order to become comfortable in assisting the patient and the family in a situation that each individual will have to face. Stage I may occur during the first three months of working with terminally ill patients.

The care providers in Stage II experience trauma, guilt, frustration, and sadness. Trauma is a major ingredient due to the need for shortened goals, and is an emotional reaction care providers experience as they relate to the reality of the dying patients' situations. They also feel frustration when they realize that the patient is going to die, that the health care team, no matter how competent, cannot prevent the death of the patient. They experience sadness when they begin to cope with their own future situations and to face the stark truth that they too will die. In addition, the process of mourning and grieving for their self and their own demise suddenly become a point at issue, a matter of life and death with them at an emotional level and on an emotional basis. This is the *Survival Stage,* and Stage I passes into Stage II involving the next three to six months.

Stage III involves further pain, mourning, and grieving. *Depression* is the noticeable element. It is the most crucial of all of the stages in learning to cope with death and dying. The care providers experience the impact of death in Stage III in different ways. Understanding this differentiation is essential. Some care providers experience extreme anxiety, grief, and depression. They question their usefulness, and their ability to contribute and to be helpful. They express anger, hurt, and self-questioning. They often speak of their "inability to come to grips with the situation." This is also the time for the care providers to "Grow or Go." In this period of growth, development, experiential and behavior sequences, mastery of self is a challenge. There is a beginning acceptance of death and an orientation to the reality of death and dying. Care providers in this stage begin to come to grips with what they will do about working with dying patients as contrasted with what they "shall do." If they are still in the "shall" mode then the possibility of going or leaving is still a part of their dynamic-ego-psyche structure. The "will" concept is needed for movement and is the forerunner of the emotional advancement towards the next stage, with a time frame of six to nine months.

At about one year, Stage IV, *Emotional Arrival,* is achieved. This involves a sense of self-protection and productive behavior with external realities moving towards internal realities. Thus, there is moderation and mitigation in relation to the sense of loss. Accommodation takes place as well as ego mastery.

When care providers feel like a helping human being, a kind of healthy interaction takes place in their personhood. The key factor is the care providers' ability to work with, on behalf of, and for the dying patient. These activities and skills may or may not be new, but the care providers are free from the constant and deep-seated emotional concern about their own death and dying. Their knowledge, skills, and human caring competencies are able to come to the surface and express themselves in behavior and performance. The learning, assimilating, emotional articulating, understanding, accepting, and adjusting of the psyche and soma have taken place. The care providers no longer need to imagine or feel that they, too, may be suffering from the same illness as the patient, and there is a moving away from identification with the patient's symptomatology.

This emotional freedom, however, in no way makes the care providers feel any less concern about the patient. It is easier for them emotionally to take hold and to let go. The hurts are less frequent, and less time is required for getting over the deaths of patients. These are important ingredients in the growth and development process as accommodation and ego mastery give impetus to the role, position, and professional stances that the care providers are able to assume. The ego masters fears, anxieties, trauma, mourning, grieving, and depression, each of which may have blocked the care providers' ability to meet the needs of dying patients and their families.

In Stage V, which is also the *Stage of Deep Compassion,* self-realization, self-awareness, and self-actualization are strong component parts. The developmental process involves the care providers doing for themselves. The growth process must contain all the elements of Stages I, II, III, and IV, plus self-actualization, and accepting illness and death realistically. The care providers have witnessed the treatment and management of the disease processes, and they have seen heroic medical and surgical procedures. They now know, and can accept, that in some instances living can be more painful than dying, both for the patient and the family. In this stage, care providers develop ways in which to move, fittingly, between self and patients and to engage with the patients in a meaningful way.

Stage V gives further evidence of the fact that learning, growth and development did take place. The ability to serve another human being and to be able to give of one's self provides evidence of the care providers' humanity to others. In addition, the care providers' behavior and performance are enhanced by the dignity and self-respect they feel. This enables them, in turn, to give dignity and respect to the dying patient. The deep compassion felt by the care providers toward the dying patient is translated into constructive and appropriate activities based on a human and professional assessment of the needs of the dying patient and the family. Without the development of the skills in Stages III and IV, Stage V cannot be reached. It occurs after one to two years of professional experience.

I would now add a sixth stage called *Inner Knowledge and Wisdom.* In Stage VI inner power and inner strength are the demonstrative attributes. Another way of stating it is this: in order to use what you know, you must know what you use. Thus, Stage VI is reflective of the doer. It is characterized by the mature, seasoned professional who operates, acts, and reacts on the basis of maturity. Mature adults are well aware of self–where they have been, where they want to go, and what they need to do to get there. This may involve further training, studying, supervision, and networking.

The burned-out syndrome is not a point at issue. Seasoned health professionals are able to prevent burn-out because they take each stage and each phase of growth and development in stride and grow in the process. They are able to identify with the terrible events and diseases of patients without getting burned-out or letting these events destroy them. Acceptance, competence, and trust are also exhibited in Stage VI. Reaching this level usually involves several years beyond Stage V, and may require eight or ten years of work and experience.

As doers, the hospice professional and the caregiver have learned, received, heard, and seen empowering experiences. They become doers of their profession, doers of society, doers of the community, and doers on the world scene. As doers, their minds are open to new ideas. They meet each day with confidence and look forward to learning, to expanding their world through knowledge and using their wisdom. Thus, they are well adjusted and secure in working in the area of death and dying.

The doers are teachers, and they share their knowledge. They know, and can do, and they do it. They bring to each situation—be it patient, family, significant other, colleague, co-worker, supervisor, community, or nation—a depth of understanding and compassion and the ability to communicate feelings. There is a freedom that comes with Stage VI. It is observable through behavior and demeanor. They find fulfillment in their work. Their lives are transformed, the higher purposes in life are obtained and their self-spirit flows from within the heart reflecting love, caring, and compassion. Therefore, they are able to cope comfortably with the pain and suffering of their fellow men, women, and children.

Underlying this entire growth and development process is an increasing level of comfort and ability in working with dying patients. The line of comfort-ability becomes the linkage between the dying patients and the care providers. It is the life-line which the care providers are able to use as part of the coping mechanism in working with dying patients. In hospice, it is the foundation of ethical, humane practice.

NOTE

1. I have addressed these areas in *Death: The Coping Mechanism of the Health Professional*, 2nd Rev. ed. (Greenville, SC: Swiger Associates, 1994).

Hospice Organizations' Role in Health Care Improvement

Sarah J. Goodlin

SUMMARY. Hospice organizations must understand and plan for their position in the proposed and ongoing changes in health care delivery in the United States. This paper proposes that hospice organizations shift their thinking about their role in the health care system. Hospices may view their work as processes which are impacted by many entities within the system of care; measure the outcomes of this work against the needs of patients, families and health care providers; and work to continually improve care. Aspects of this approach, and its implications for hospice organizations, are described. Using this new understanding, hospice organizations can both broaden their impact on care for larger numbers of dying patients, and position themselves to move forward within that system as the financial base and structure of health care change. *[Article copies available for a fee from The Haworth Document Delivery Service: 1-800-342-9678. E-mail address: getinfo@haworth.com]*

Hospice programs in the United States arose as grass roots movements to provide an alternative to traditional health care for dying patients. The

Sarah J. Goodlin, MD, is Assistant Professor of Medicine, Dartmouth Medical School and Associate Chief of Staff for Geriatrics and Extended Care at the White River Junction Veterans Administration Medical Center.

Address correspondence to: Sarah J. Goodlin, MD, Geriatrics and Extended Care (11B), White River Junction Veterans Administration Medical Center, White River Junction, VT 05009.

Dr. Goodlin is a Faculty Scholar, Open Society Institute, Project on Death in America.

[Haworth co-indexing entry note]: "Hospice Organizations' Role in Health Care Improvement." Goodlin, Sarah J. Co-published simultaneously in *The Hospice Journal* (The Haworth Press, Inc.) Vol. 12, No. 2, 1997, pp. 71-80; and: *Ethics in Hospice Care: Challenges to Hospice Values in a Changing Health Care Environment* (ed: Bruce Jennings) The Haworth Press, Inc., 1997, pp. 71-80. Single or multiple copies of this article are available for a fee from The Haworth Document Delivery Service [1-800-342-9678, 9:00 a.m. - 5:00 p.m. (EST). E-mail address: getinfo@haworth.com].

development of the Medicare and insurance "hospice benefit" financially intertwined hospice programs with the rest of medical care. Hospice organizations face financial and ethical challenges in the proposed and ongoing changes in healthcare delivery in the United States. Structural and financial changes, regulation and standardization of practice, and public demands for value and accountability simultaneously confront health care providers. How do hospice organizations sort amongst these challenges to plan for the future? How well does hospice care meet patients' needs? How do patients, payers, and others assess the value and quality of care provided? How can we show that hospice work is valuable? How can we provide support and time-intensive care to patients and their families while controlling costs? What role does hospice play in the system of care for patients nearing the end of life?

Tools and knowledge gained from business and industry, such as systems thinking and continual improvement, offer a means of understanding and planning for hospice's position in this turbulent period in health care. Systems thinking shifts the way we see what we do: work is a process which is impacted by many entities within a system of care, and whose outcomes can be measured. The process is driven by the needs of those who receive services: patients, families, and other health care providers. Viewing health care as a system clarifies the relationships and interactions between health care providers, patients, and others who supply the process, do the work in the process, and benefit from the outcomes of the process. "Quality Improvement" or "Continual Improvement" uses basic concepts which are also at the foundation of hospice work:

- "Patient-centered" work: focusing the care on needs of patients and families, and others in the health care system who benefit from hospice services
- monitoring and evaluating the outcomes of work
- continually trying to improve care.

This paper will review methods which can facilitate growth and learning within hospice organizations, and tools through which an understanding of how the relationships and interface between hospice and others in the health care system can work to enhance care for a broad spectrum of patients.

HOSPICE'S POSITION IN THE HEALTH CARE SYSTEM

The medical knowledge base in palliative care has grown substantially, yet dying patients often suffer physically, emotionally, and spiritually.

Hospice has succeeded in providing an alternative to usual medical care, focusing on patient and family needs, and on quality of life for the patient and family. Yet, there may be many additional patients who would benefit from hospice care. Could hospice organizations serve individuals who do not routinely access hospice care? Can similar care be provided to those not enrolled in hospice? Those referred to hospice on average receive hospice services for only the final month of their lives. Should hospice services be provided earlier in the course of care? Should hospice integrate into healthcare at large, to increase the number of individuals who benefit from hospice services or philosophy? How can the knowledge and skills of hospice care for dying patients be integrated into the training of new nurses and physicians? An answer to these questions may come from clarifying the position of hospice within the local health care system, and improving care for dying patients within the system as a whole.

An analogy used to explain "systems thinking" is that of the three blindfolded people who come upon an elephant. Each describes the elephant from the perspective of the body part nearest them (the leg, the tail or the trunk), and none appreciates the entire elephant, the relationship of their part to the whole, or the function of the elephant, until they communicate with each other to form a composite image, or better, remove their blindfolds to see the elephant, and watch it move and eat.

While not organized as such in most communities, there is a system within the greater system of health care which provides care for patients near the end of life. This system includes physicians, local hospitals, nursing homes, community-based long term care agencies, formal and informal community supports, religious organizations, and others. As the components of this system clarify their relationships to others, they can develop a common sense of purpose, and can more effectively work to improve quality of life for dying patients. Aspects of hospice care, including a focus on patient and family needs, clear goals for palliation, and tools to perform assessments and monitor symptoms and problems, can be integrated into the health care system's approach to care. Service providers can understand both their own role and how they function together to produce relief from symptoms, support for emotional and existential reconciliation, and enhanced quality of life for dying patients and their families. Understanding how different parts of the health care system function together to meet patients' and others' needs can reduce variation in care, avoid duplication of services, and enhance utilization of resources.

Development of a common purpose and approach to care within the health care system creates a continuum of care for dying patients that can effectively integrate hospice philosophy and skills in multiple settings, including acute care and training institutions. Knowledge of, and planning within, the system of care for dying patients will position hospice organizations to move through the turbulent restructuring of health care.

IMPROVING CARE

The approach of improving care outlined in Figure 1 can enhance the work of each individual in the organization. Hospice providers become aware of how well they personally, and the system, meet needs by documenting patient outcomes such as effectiveness of symptom management, physical independence, spiritual support, and outcomes for physicians and other providers such as effectiveness of communication, or the extent to which hospice facilitates the work of these other providers. From this data, hospice providers can also begin to understand how those they serve attach value to what they do. Value is a complicated subjective concept, which includes how "good" something is, usually relative to its "cost." Value is enhanced by optimizing outcomes, while simultaneously minimizing, or not increasing, costs. Clarifying needs, priorities and value focuses everyone's work, and helps set organization goals for service. Continually reevaluating and improving work, its outcomes, and the process by which it is accomplished brings insight and excitement to work.

PROCESS OF CARE

To improve care effectively, organizations need to understand how that care is provided, and how they interact with others in delivering care. Much of the understanding of a system of healthcare depends upon understanding the provision of healthcare as a process. That is, there are a series of steps in providing care to meet a certain need. Hospice organizations provide care and support to dying patients and their families. Simulta-

FIGURE 1. Steps in the Improvement of Care

- clarify needs and priorities of those served by hospice,
- understand the outcomes and process of care,
- identify points at which care can be improved,
- design improvements,
- implement improvements,
- evaluate the outcomes of the improved process.

neously, they serve physicians and acute hospitals by assisting in their care of dying patients. These are two separate but related processes, designed to meet different needs with definable outcomes. Hospice organizations have defined explicit steps in the care and support of patients and families, with tools to assess symptoms and problems and to monitor the effectiveness of interventions.

The steps in that process (assess–intervene–monitor effect–modify intervention) are fairly easy to identify. Other processes in the work of hospice, such as assisting physicians and hospitals to care for patients, may be less obvious, but are most likely also well developed (accept referral–assess patient–report findings–recommend intervention, and so on). The steps in a process can be defined by "talking" a health care provider, or the patient and family, through their experience: "How does the care begin? What happens next? And then what? . . . ". The primary work of caring for dying patients, or "core" process, is clarified by identifying the basic steps necessary to the provision of care. As such, it represents the desired process of care, and can be compared to the current (or actual) process of care–steps patients currently go through to receive care. The comparison of current care with optimal care identifies gaps between the two, and areas of significant variation in care, where improvements might be made. Once we identify the process, then we can evaluate how well what we do meets the needs of and enhances outcomes for those we serve.

Figure 2 is a draft of a core process for "Palliative Care" developed as part of a quality improvement effort in our community (The Upper Valley of the Connecticut river, in Vermont and New Hampshire). Supporting processes, such as education, communication, and financing, impact care throughout the core process. The steps in the core process are the basic hospice approach to care. However, in our community, these steps are not consistently a part of care for patients who die outside of hospice. Making the steps explicit allows members of the improvement team to understand the steps, and gain insight into how and where current care can be improved.

In our local improvement efforts, for example, comparison of current care to our "core process" yielded many opportunities for improvement:

- *Explicit goals of care.* While routine in hospice care, this step occurred infrequently in outpatient and acute inpatient settings. When the goals of care were outlined, these goals were not clearly recorded for all care providers to review. Uncertainty about the goals and plan of care resulted in mixed messages about care, inadequate symptom relief, and in the patient undergoing unnecessary procedures or tests.

- *Explicit plan of care.* In acute and skilled long term care, the plan of care was not reformulated and recorded once it was recognized that the patient was dying and wished palliative interventions only.
- *Referrals to hospice and other resources.* Referrals from outpatient, inpatient, and community-based care to hospice and other resources for care in non-hospital settings occur without an organized approach.
- *Education.* Patients and families are not educated through a defined process.

MEASUREMENT OF QUALITY

How can hospice providers know how well they satisfy the needs of patients, families, and physicians, and other health care workers, hospitals, and social service agencies with whom they interact? Initially, the system must clarify the needs of patients, families and others. The concepts of needs and of value are intertwined with preferences for care, and with the understanding by patients and families of the potential benefits and burdens of various medical interventions and therapies, and the limitations of medicine. If the limitations of medical care, and the benefits and burdens of various options are clear, patients and their families may be able to be clear about their expectations and preferences. Outcomes of care near the end of life can be defined by the satisfaction of patient and family needs, physical parameters (such as minimal pain or dyspnea), patient function (physical, social, emotional and spiritual), and cost. Other sets of outcomes are based on how well hospice services meet the needs of others in the health care community in satisfactorily providing care to these patients. How patients and the community judge the value of the services produced (that is, how "good" is the service, and how good is it relative to its cost?) may be impacted by other factors. These, as well as perceived needs, can be assessed by hospice and other health care providers by asking patients and their families what is important to them, and what they value and need.

Family members' perceptions of pain, suffering, and need may differ significantly from patients' perceptions. It is important to prospectively clarify both the patient's and family's symptoms and values to tailor interventions to meet their individual needs. Tracking how well hospice services meet specific needs (caregiver support, emotional support for the patient, management of pain and other symptoms, easing the delivery of care for physicians) on an individual-patient basis can provide insight into what is done well and what needs to improve. Moreover, because these

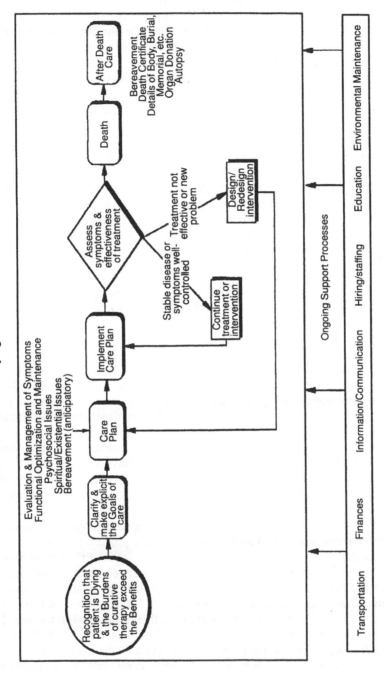

FIGURE 2. Care of Dying Patients: Core Process

data have yet to be reported in the literature, compiling this information can help the medical community identify measures of value and quality for end of life care. Measures of quality which are multifactorial, incorporating measures of physical outcomes, function, satisfaction relative to need, and value, can help us strategically plan for improvements in the quality and value of work, and measure the success of interventions. Measurement of performance against these quality factors can be integrated into usual work, so that it becomes clear that the focus of work is to better meet the needs of patients, families and other health care providers.

In the face of increasing regulation and standardization of healthcare, it is important that hospice organizations, and others directly involved in caring for patients at the end of life, develop these measures of quality and value. Without insight from direct assessment of patient and family needs, regulatory or other bodies may assign some measure to end of life care which misses the essence of patient-centered palliative care.

HOW CAN DEFINING THE PROCESS
OF CARE BENEFIT HOSPICE?

The cost of care and quality of care are unavoidably tied to the process of care. The process of care provides insight into the measures of quality and value of care. Improvement efforts can focus on streamlining the process of care, on reducing variation in care, or on closing the gap between current care and optimal care. All of these efforts can improve the outcomes of care and better meet the needs of patients and the community.

Hospice's role in the process of providing care near the end of life can be made explicit. Knowledge and skills of hospice staff can contribute to the definition of the process of care, and thus have a broad impact on the care of dying patients in multiple venues. Making explicit the components of the core process, understanding how they can be accomplished, and who is responsible for them increases understanding among providers and staff about their work. Clarifying the plan of care provides education to others about this care. Application of the core process to different venues can reduce the variation in care for patients dying in different settings.

Specific improvement efforts can enhance communication between hospice and the other participants in the health care system. For example, the palliative care core process begins with "Recognition that the patient is dying and that the burdens of curative therapy outweigh the benefits." This point alone may influence the timeliness of referrals to hospice; if either recognition that the patient is dying or a decision that the burdens of aggressive therapy outweigh the benefits come late in an individual's illness, then hospice referrals will occur shortly before death. Understanding the components of this first step may allow hospice team members to work with members of their healthcare system to refer patients to hospice earlier in their care. Clear and explicit goals for care, and a plan of care, enhance communication and provision of care for dying patients across many settings.

Measuring the outcome of work in terms of how well hospice programs and others meet the needs of patients, families and other health care providers can strengthen hospice's position in the structure of the health care system. If this measurement includes assessments of the impact of the work on improving function, reducing suffering and supporting the patient and family, in addition to "satisfaction," we may be able to shift the focus of care for dying patients in other health care organizations to these important outcomes. Monitors of cost in dollars to the patient and family and to insurers, as well as indirect costs to the patient and others, will be necessary to guide decisions about the need for certain types of care. The integration of measurement of outcomes, followed by improvement trials and reassessment, into patient care will broaden knowledge within the hospice organization and within the larger healthcare system, and should help us focus care on those things which are really important to patients.

In addition, streamlining care can conserve scarce resources and improve the value of the work done by hospice and others. Evaluation of the process of care usually results in a reduction in the cost of care. Significant variation in care has been identified as a cause of expense, as well as a cause of variable quality of care. Evaluation of and reduction in variation in health care delivery results in the streamlining of care, and in doing so reduces cost.

CONCLUSION

Understanding the provision of health care for patients nearing the end of life as a system, and hospice's position in that system, will enable hospice organizations to improve relationships with other components of the care system. Needs of the community and of patients and families can be identified clearly. Defining the process of care for dying patients can establish a framework for evaluating that care, clarifying outcomes, measuring value, and reducing costs. The provision of care can be improved within the context of this system. In working to understand and improve care, hospice organizations can both broaden their impact on care for larger numbers of dying patients, and position themselves to move forward within that system as the financial base and structure of health care change.

REFERENCES

Batalden PB, Stoltz PK, "A Framework for the Continual Improvement of Health Care: Building and Applying Professional and Improvement Knowledge to Test Changes in Daily Work," *Joint Commission Journal on Quality Improvement* 19 (10): 424-445, 1993.

Blumenthal D, Scheck A, Eds. *Improving Clinical Practice,* San Francisco: Jossey-Bass, 1995.

Hospice and Managed Care

John J. Mahoney

SUMMARY. Managed care is having a significant effect on the delivery of hospice care. A primary concern facing hospices is that reimbursement rates will likely either remain stable or fall. This suggests that competition between health care networks will lead to mergers and the closing of some hospices. A second challenge is the immense pressure to make decisions based exclusively on the cost/benefit ratio of hospice in a context where managed care organizations seek to increase market share and improve profits. To foster good hospice care within a managed care environment, service providers need to be defined, criteria for referral to hospice programs must be crafted, payments should be based on a per diem method, benefit packages should identify a comprehensive package of services, and agreements between hospices and managed care organizations should allow for routine review and amendments to their contracts. *[Article copies available for a fee from The Haworth Document Delivery Service: 1-800-342-9678. E-mail address: getinfo@haworth.com]*

Whether one believes that the inexorable march to embrace managed care is the long-awaited answer to the ever-increasing cost of health care, a politically necessary stepping stone to a "single-payer" system, or marking-of-time while emerging provider networks learn the financial intricacies of direct contracting and risk-sharing, one must agree that managed care is having a profound effect on the entire health care community,

John J. Mahoney is the President of the National Hospice Organization.

Address correspondence to: John J. Mahoney, National Hospice Organization, 1901 N. Moore Street, Suite 901, Arlington, VA 22209.

[Haworth co-indexing entry note]: "Hospice and Managed Care." Mahoney, John J. Co-published simultaneously in *The Hospice Journal* (The Haworth Press, Inc.) Vol. 12, No. 2, 1997, pp. 81-84; and: *Ethics in Hospice Care: Challenges to Hospice Values in a Changing Health Care Environment* (ed: Bruce Jennings) The Haworth Press, Inc., 1997, pp. 81-84. Single or multiple copies of this article are available for a fee from The Haworth Document Delivery Service [1-800-342-9678, 9:00 a.m. - 5:00 p.m. (EST). E-mail address: getinfo@haworth.com].

including hospice care. The private marketplace has already made a significant commitment to providing health care through managed care companies, and recent proposals currently working their way through the legislative process will, over time, change the Medicare and Medicaid programs from primarily fee-for-service to managed care programs.

Such changes to the traditional methods of paying for hospice care have caused alarm in the hospice community. Such alarm, while perhaps overstated, is not completely unwarranted. Still, the move towards managed care should be viewed by hospices primarily as an opportunity.

Historically, Managed Care Organizations (MCOs) have not met the needs of terminally ill persons any more effectively or economically than traditional forms of health care. As interdisciplinary team-based care, guided by a single plan of care, hospice is already managed care. Also, under the current per diem payment methodology of Medicare and Medicaid, hospice care has more than a decade of experience in sharing financial risk with the payer of health care. Such knowledge and experience will make hospice care a valued partner within the networks of managed care providers. For hospices, such partnerships could allow greater access to hospice care.

The primary concern that hospices face is the realization that under a predominantly managed care system, reimbursement will not continue to rise at the current rate, and may even fall. Such reductions will occur even though for some hospices, particularly in more rural areas, current reimbursement from Medicare and Medicaid does not fully cover the cost of care to beneficiaries. Another concern is that as competition increases between the various networks, it is probable that increasing numbers of hospices will merge, creating larger programs. This process will be most likely to develop in communities where there are large numbers of hospice programs relative to the population. Such consolidation could prove most painful to those hospices with long histories of community involvement and support.

In spite of such concerns, the partnership between hospice and managed care is a natural one with benefits for both, but it will not develop without the ongoing efforts of hospice executives.

Currently, MCOs are consumed by the need to increase market share, manage the challenges of merging organizations, and as many are now for-profit organizations they must also focus on profit margins in the face of flat or declining premium growth per member. Such challenges can leave MCO executives with little inclination to explore new services, regardless of the potential benefits.

In addressing this challenge of bringing the benefits of hospice care to the attention of MCOs, hospices would do well to focus on several critical points. Even though there will be significant pressure to focus almost exclusively on the cost benefits of hospice care, that is not necessarily the most critical component of a successful partnership:

- Hospice is the most appropriate form of care for the terminally ill. With an emphasis on palliative medicine, including a specific focus on pain management and symptom control, hospice care also addresses the patient's psychosocial and spiritual needs.
- Hospice is managed care. Under a single plan of care, hospice provides services across a continuum of locations, e.g., the patient's personal residence, an inpatient setting, or a group residence such as a nursing home.
- Hospice cares for the patient and the family. Attention to the concerns of the family could lessen their future health care needs.
- Health care at the end of life consumes a disproportionate share of health care dollars. Hospice providers have more than a decade of sharing the cost risks related to providing health care to the terminally ill with the payers of health care. By sharing the cost risk of such care with a hospice, the MCO can more easily define its risk and budget accordingly.
- Hospice care is a comprehensive set of services. People in need of end-of-life care do not want the additional burden of coordinating care between multiple providers, even if the providers are in the same provider network. No other provider brings to the patient's home a more complete set of services.
- Hospice care can reduce the cost of health care through the substitution of care in the home versus hospitalizations.

Beyond the obstacles that hospice programs will need to overcome to make MCOs aware of the benefits of hospice care are the challenges inherent in establishing contractual relationships with MCOs that are fair and reasonable to the MCO's members (and potential hospice patients), the MCO itself, and the hospice program. Several items that should be considered part of a well-structured, mutually-beneficial agreement include:

- Definition of service provider. Only licensed, certified or accredited hospices should be part of the relationship.
- Payment to the hospice should be based on a per diem method. In the future, enough cost data and payment history with MCOs will be developed, allowing alternative payment methodologies to be ex-

plored. Currently, neither the hospice or the MCO (including consulting actuaries) have sufficient data to craft alternatives, including per member capitation contracts.

- The benefit package should identify a comprehensive package of services similar to the current Medicare Hospice Benefit. The provision of such services as inpatient care, pharmaceuticals and durable medical equipment (DME) can be negotiable depending on the MCO's relationships with these other providers. Even though other providers may be delivering certain services to the terminally ill patient, the hospice must be required to maintain overall patient management and responsibility. Arrangements using other providers for certain services could allow flexibility in negotiating per-diem rates.

- Criteria for referral to the hospice program must be carefully crafted and made part of the contract to eliminate incentives for inappropriate referral to the hospice.

- The agreement between the hospice and the MCO should include a provision allowing for routine review and amendment to the contract in order to maintain the agreement in a fair and equitable manner.

The health care environment is changing at a pace that few could have predicted. Hospice care is very much a part of that change. Despite the challenges, partnerships between hospices and managed care companies will be critical to the continued expansion of access to hospice care and to insuring the availability of hospice care to those in need for the foreseeable future.

The Future of Hospice in a Reformed American Health Care System: What Are the Real Questions?

Larry Beresford

SUMMARY. Many supporters of the hospice movement are concerned about changes being imposed on the movement by market-based reforms in the larger health care industry. But if they are to truly encourage the preservation of hospice's core goals and values in caring for vulnerable patients with terminal illnesses, they need to understand the realities of day-to-day hospice care under today's managed care system. The future of hospice in America will not be determined by its tax status or administrative structure, but by its functional integration into new systems of care, flexibility in response to emerging terminal care needs, commitment to standards and measurable quality outcomes and clearer articulation of the value an appropriately financed hospice movement can offer to patients at the end of their lives. *[Article copies available for a fee from The Haworth Document Delivery Service: 1-800-342-9678. E-mail address: getinfo@haworth.com]*

Larry Beresford is a San Francisco-based independent health care journalist; writer/editor of the *Hospice Manager's Monograph* and of the *Hospice News Service,* a monthly news source for state hospice organizations; and contributor to *Hospice Magazine,* Faulkner & Gray's *Medicine & Health Perspectives* and *Health Plan Magazine.*

Address correspondence to: Larry Beresford, P.O. Box 31516, San Francisco, CA 94131.

[Haworth co-indexing entry note]: "The Future of Hospice in a Reformed American Health Care System: What Are the Real Questions?" Beresford, Larry. Co-published simultaneously in *The Hospice Journal* (The Haworth Press, Inc.) Vol. 12, No. 2, 1997, pp. 85-91; and: *Ethics in Hospice Care: Challenges to Hospice Values in a Changing Health Care Environment* (ed: Bruce Jennings) The Haworth Press, Inc., 1997, pp. 85-91. Single or multiple copies of this article are available for a fee from The Haworth Document Delivery Service [1-800-342-9678, 9:00 a.m. - 5:00 p.m. (EST). E-mail address: getinfo@haworth.com].

Sandol Stoddard, in her classic 1978 book on the hospice movement, sums up the challenges facing the Hospice of Marin County, CA, Board of Directors at their meeting on November 11, 1976, with the following question: "How then to organize properly, without losing touch with the *esprit* that has already developed? The spirit is strong—stronger than ever, now that Hospice of Marin has shown what it can do. But the flesh is weary, and local banks have a way of reminding people rather regularly when their accounts are overdrawn. . . . No one here really wants to talk about money, but under the circumstances, money in quantity has become a necessity" (Stoddard 1978).

While the specific issues confronting the American hospice movement have changed since those early days, the bedrock challenge remains the same: how to preserve the movement's essential values of compassion and commitment to the real needs of dying patients in the face of growth, financial imperatives and the potential corrupting influence of money.

A CNN-TV News Update broadcast on May 30, 1995, described an "unlikely partnership" between "compassionate hospices" and "cost-conscious" managed care organizations. "Hospice's mission of mercy is generally provided on a not-for-profit basis," CNN reporter Jeff Levine said, but "that's changing as hospice carves out a niche in the bottom-line world of managed care" (Video Monitoring Services of America, Inc. 1995).

For some who have admired the movement from arm's length, the marriage of hospice and managed care may seem incongruous. Others ask analogous questions: how did this idealistic, mission-driven movement become a $1.5 to $2 billion industry with over 2,500 providers nationwide, some of them multi-million-dollar operations employing hundreds of full-time staff? The industry's fastest growing sector is profit-making, entrepreneurial hospices, yet proprietary hospice care is still viewed by many as an oxymoron. The classic image, conveyed by Stoddard's work and others, is of small, volunteer, spiritually inspired, caring communities helping highly motivated individuals on their ultimate journey of self-discovery. But this image seems to be receding ever farther from the routines of today's hospices, while some front-line hospice professionals even question whether such an image is still relevant to the needs of terminally ill patients.

Such concerns about growth and change in the poorly understood hospice movement are also present in the professional literature. Two prominent recent examples reflect this international dialogue. James and Field (1992) discuss the "routinization" of a "charismatic," formerly separatist hospice movement, arguing that any such movement inevitably becomes bureaucratized. A survey of Australian hospice nurses proposes to examine the threat of institutionalization for hospice's "Good Death ideal" (McNamara et al. 1994).

America's hospice providers, always eager for the opportunity to share their stories of compassionate engagement with the realities of terminal illness that most people would rather not contemplate, are grateful for the attention. They welcome any public scrutiny that could aid them in doing the best and most skilled job possible in fulfilling their mission of caring for vulnerable dying patients.

But are hospice's well-meaning supporters asking the wrong questions? Does a lack of general awareness about the way hospice care works in the context of today's market-based health care reform, along with an overly romanticized image of the "good death," divert needed attention from the real issues now confronting the American hospice movement? How, for instance, could hospices possibly avoid becoming intimately involved with managed care, when managed care is becoming the dominant health care payment mechanism, not just in the private sector but very likely soon for Medicare and Medicaid as well? How could they hope to provide their skilled, labor-intensive, interdisciplinary professional management of terminal symptoms for significant numbers of patients without access to payment from health insurers, and why should they have to?

It is important for hospice's current and potential allies to understand these day-to-day realities, if they are to encourage the preservation of hospice's core goals and values. Experienced hospice managers recognize that there is no longer a question of whether hospice care in America will go through tremendous transformations in response to changes in the larger health care system. The more relevant question is whether established providers might be able to influence the direction of those changes and how much of hospice's essential philosophy might survive. Some of the ways that essence is being challenged today include the following:

Managed care's commitment to wring waste out of health expenditures will put pressures on hospices, especially if, as predicted, managed care contracts are awarded primarily on the basis of price discounts. A related problem is how to make payers understand–and cover–hospice's interdisciplinary, all-inclusive, mini-managed-care approach to coordinating the services required by terminally ill patients. This combined medical, psychosocial and supportive service package may not jibe with the models of cost management now being developed by managed care payors. They may only be willing to pay for certain aspects of the holistic hospice package, such as nurse or physician services.

The development of integrated health delivery systems challenges hospices to understand these new networks and how to claim a niche in them. If physicians and other health providers under capitation become contractually constrained in the referrals they can make, existing hospices might be frozen out. Nor does it make sense for hospices to be isolated from these comprehensive systems as they assemble integrated, cradle-to-grave continuums of health care for covered populations.

The landscape of hospice providers is also changing rapidly, with the growth of national for-profit chains, investor groups and contract management firms as well as the development of hospice "product lines" by huge national hospital, nursing home, home care and high-tech corporations. It is also changing due to increased competition for referrals in many cities between hospices and with home health agencies offering terminal care or cancer care alternatives.

Meanwhile, the caseload served by hospices has changed considerably from the movement's origins in suburban communities and largely white, middle-class, stable-family populations. The ravages of terminal illness, requiring the specialized support of hospice, affect a much broader cross section of Americans, but notions of acceptance (as defined by Elisabeth Kubler-Ross) or of the "good death" may not translate easily across cultural boundaries. Leading hospice managers increasingly notice that many of their "customers" or potential customers are intimidated by or unreceptive to the hospice concept as they perceive it. This is spurring the development of "pre-hospice" or special care services for those who, regardless of the clinical evidence, are unwilling or unable to acknowledge even the possibility that their illness might be terminal. Others have developed new models, definitions and service packages to care for people with HIV disease or Alzheimer's.

Instead of judging hospice providers by their tax or administrative status or the source of their funding, we should be working toward clear, reliable and valid ways of measuring and evaluating each hospice to ensure that it is delivering comprehensive, coordinated, expert, individualized care addressing each patient's physical, emotional, psychological, social and spiritual symptoms of terminal illness. Here are some other issues to consider in terms of preserving hospice values in the face of change.

- How will standards of quality hospice care be defined, whether through licensure, accreditation or peer review, and who will enforce them? External monitors such as the Joint Commission on Accreditation of Healthcare Organizations can only enforce minimum standards. Who, then, will define comparative optimal standards? What are the minimum and optimal level of staffing and other services?

Professional competencies? Where are hospice's benchmarking standards? What are the objective yardsticks to differentiate quality hospice providers, regardless of tax status, from profiteers?

- What are quantifiable outcomes measures in hospice, given that the mortality rate is nearly 100 percent? How do we meaningfully define and measure quality of life in people whose functional status is in precipitous decline?

- What are the core values, goals and guiding mission of hospice? For example, while hospice was never in the business of *telling* patients the best way to die, how can providers better balance the tension between promoting patient autonomy and offering guidance about what can be achieved at this difficult time? Can the movement articulate and communicate its bedrock goals as many of its traditional trappings and structures fall away under health care reform?

- Are there effective new methods of defining and pricing hospice's package of services, for example, under capitation? What will be the impact of the predicted passing of the Medicare model of hospice reimbursement and the expansion of hospice services beyond the customary population of patients with a prognosis of six months or less to live? Will new models of "pre-hospice" jeopardize hospice's identity as a program of care for the dying?

- Who will provide hospice care? Who will be their health care partners? Where does hospice care fit into integrated delivery systems? Who will teach the new corporate hospice professionals, who have come to the field for a job, not a mission, about the spirit that drove the movement's founders?

What, ultimately, is special about hospice, and how can we articulate it for all concerned in order to preserve it? Thousands of surviving family members of hospice patients express gratitude for the support that helped them not only to cope with the most traumatic crisis of their lives but even turn it into a positive experience of personal growth. However, the movement needs a language for communicating these small miracles that happen every day in hospice. Is the hospice experience ultimately a matter only of symptom management, broadly and holistically defined, or is there something more to be said about the confrontation with mortality that happens under hospice's care?[1] And if so, how can it be transmitted to payors, referral sources, regulators, consumers and the public?

The answers to these questions are tremendously important, for a number of reasons. Consider that an estimated 1.2 million Americans will be diagnosed with cancer this year. Despite continuing advances in cancer treatment, nearly half will die from their disease, often with the pain, discomfort and psychosocial distress that hospice care is designed to relieve. The growing elderly population will experience increased rates of other chronic, degenerative diseases that cannot be cured. And following behind is the Baby Boomer generation, now confronting the simultaneous realities of elderly parents and inklings of its own mortality at a time when limits on what health care can achieve are finally becoming clearer.

Hospice's cost-effectiveness was demonstrated anew in a recent study showing that Medicare saved $1.52 for every dollar it spent on hospice care (Lewin-VHI, Inc. 1995). But this demonstration of cost-effectiveness was achieved in a medical system that paid for both hospice and conventional care alternatives. Hospice's cost-effectiveness thus is predicated on adequate funding, in order to appropriately and preventively manage the symptoms of illness and support families to cope and continue playing an important role in the patient's care—thereby minimizing crises, emergency room visits and hospital stays.

Hospice may not be less costly than institutional neglect or an approach by insurers of pushing dying patients out of hospitals and onto their own scant resources. Nor is it less costly, in purely financial terms, than legalized physician-assisted suicide or a policy of urging terminally ill patients to check out early—in order to spare them and the system the "hassles" of terminal care. The true quality of life in the face of disease's ravages that is possible in hospice must be communicated, and it must be valued, if it is to be preserved. Ultimately, the challenges now facing the hospice movement can only be answered in a context of what our society is willing to pay to relieve the suffering of those with terminal illnesses and to help them live out their lives in ways that are meaningful to them.

NOTE

1. For example, hospice physician Ira Byock, in a keynote presentation at the May 1995 National Hospice Organization Management Meeting in Washington, DC, proposed a conceptual model of preserving opportunities for patients at the end of life and of lifelong growth and development through life's final phase.

REFERENCES

James, N., and D. Field. "The Routinization of Hospice: Charisma and Bureaucratization." *Social Science and Medicine* 34(12): 1363-1375, 1992.
Lewin-VHI, Inc. *An Analysis of the Cost Savings of the Medicare Hospice Benefit.* Washington, D.C., May, 1995.

McNamara, B., C. Waddell, and M. Colvin. "The Institutionalization of the Good Death." *Social Science and Medicine* 39(11): 1501-1508, 1994.

Stoddard, S. *The Hospice Movement: A Better Way of Caring for the Dying.* Briarcliff Manor, NY: Stein and Day; 1978.

Video Monitoring Services of America, Inc., CNN-TV News Update, Washington, D.C., May 30, 1995.

Index

Access to hospice care
  current patient profile statistics, 11
  expansion of, with view toward
    diversity and potential
    barriers, 73,88
  agenda recommendations,
    15-16
  disenfranchised, displaced,
    stigmatized populations,
    12,15
  family composition, structure,
    attitudes, expectations, 11,
    12-14,15
  health care access methods,
    providers, 12
  home settings, deficient or
    non-traditional, 11,15-16
  illnesses deviant from cancer
    model, 14,15,22
    and "pre-hospice"
      services, 88,89
  religious influences, 12-13
  staffing adaptations, 12,15-16
Adkins, Janet, 22
Age of patients, 11,14
AIDS/HIV, persons with, 11,14,26,
  44,45,88
Alcoholics and drug-addicted
  persons, 12,14,44,46
ALS, persons with, 14,22
Alzheimer's, persons with, 22,88
Anxieties of care providers toward
  dying and hospice care,
  coping mechanisms for,
  66-70
Arthritis, severe, 22
Assisted suicide; physician assisted;
  legalized

  arguments for legalization, 2
  cost-effectiveness, 20,24,90
  endurance fostered via option
    of, 23
  fears and guilt, 19-20,21,23
  quality of life and dignity,
    20-21,22
  hospice survival jeopardized by,
    2,18,19,23-24
  states' legalization, 18
Autonomy of terminally ill persons
  and assisted suicide legalization
    arguments, 19,22-23
  boundaries of, 13
  hospice as haven for, 3-4,5
  nurses' ethical responsibilities
    toward, 34
  pain as threat to, 28

Beneficence and non-maleficence,
  concepts of, 34
  and principle of double effect,
    29-30
Burn-out syndrome, prevention of,
  69-70
Burns, victims of severe, 22

Cancer patients, statistics
  of pain level experiences, 26
  served by hospice, 11
Cancer, progressive terminal model,
  illnesses deviant from, as
  hospice challenges, 14,15,
  22,88,89
Caring in hospice, defined, 66
  and coping mechanisms for
    anxieties related to, 66-70